SECONDHAND SMOKE EXPOSURE AND CARDIOVASCULAR EFFECTS

Making Sense of the Evidence

Committee on Secondhand Smoke Exposure and Acute Coronary Events

Board on Population Health and Public Health Practice

INSTITUTE OF MEDICINE
OF THE NATIONAL ACADEMIES

THE NATIONAL ACADEMIES PRESS
Washington, D.C.
www.nap.edu

THE NATIONAL ACADEMIES PRESS   500 Fifth Street, N.W.   Washington, DC 20001

NOTICE: The project that is the subject of this report was approved by the Governing Board of the National Research Council, whose members are drawn from the councils of the National Academy of Sciences, the National Academy of Engineering, and the Institute of Medicine. The members of the committee responsible for the report were chosen for their special competences and with regard for appropriate balance.

This study was supported by Contract No. 200-2005-13434, TO#11 between the National Academy of Sciences and the U.S. Centers for Disease Control and Prevention. Any opinions, findings, conclusions, or recommendations expressed in this publication are those of the author(s) and do not necessarily reflect the view of the organizations or agencies that provided support for this project.

Library of Congress Cataloging-in-Publication Data

Secondhand smoke exposure and cardiovascular effects : making sense of the evidence / Committee on Secondhand Smoke Exposure and Acute Coronary Events, Board on Population Health and Public Health Practice.
    p. ; cm.
  Includes bibliographical references.
  ISBN 978-0-309-13839-0 (pbk.)
  1. Coronary heart disease—Risk factors. 2. Passive smoking—Health aspects. I. Institute of Medicine (U.S.). Committee on Secondhand Smoke Exposure and Acute Coronary Events.
  [DNLM: 1. Cardiovascular Diseases—epidemiology. 2. Cardiovascular Diseases—prevention & control. 3. Occupational Exposure—legislation & jurisprudence. 4. Smoking—legislation & jurisprudence. 5. Tobacco Smoke Pollution—adverse effects. WG 120 S445 2009]
  RA645.H4S43 2009
  616.1'2305—dc22
                                    2009049617

Additional copies of this report are available from the National Academies Press, 500 Fifth Street, N.W., Lockbox 285, Washington, DC 20055; (800) 624-6242 or (202) 334-3313 (in the Washington metropolitan area); Internet, http://www.nap.edu.

For more information about the Institute of Medicine, visit the IOM home page at www.iom.edu.

The serpent has been a symbol of long life, healing, and knowledge among almost all cultures and religions since the beginning of recorded history. The serpent adopted as a logotype by the Institute of Medicine is a relief carving from ancient Greece, now held by the Staatliche Museen in Berlin.

Suggested citation: IOM (Institute of Medicine). 2010. *Secondhand Smoke Exposure and Cardiovascular Effects: Making Sense of the Evidence*. Washington, DC: The National Academies Press.

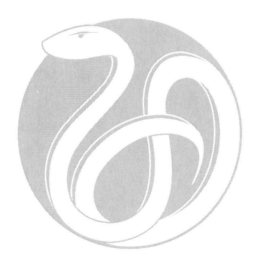

INSTITUTE OF MEDICINE
OF THE NATIONAL ACADEMIES

Advising the Nation. Improving Health.

THE NATIONAL ACADEMIES
Advisers to the Nation on Science, Engineering, and Medicine

The **National Academy of Sciences** is a private, nonprofit, self-perpetuating society of distinguished scholars engaged in scientific and engineering research, dedicated to the furtherance of science and technology and to their use for the general welfare. Upon the authority of the charter granted to it by the Congress in 1863, the Academy has a mandate that requires it to advise the federal government on scientific and technical matters. Dr. Ralph J. Cicerone is president of the National Academy of Sciences.

The **National Academy of Engineering** was established in 1964, under the charter of the National Academy of Sciences, as a parallel organization of outstanding engineers. It is autonomous in its administration and in the selection of its members, sharing with the National Academy of Sciences the responsibility for advising the federal government. The National Academy of Engineering also sponsors engineering programs aimed at meeting national needs, encourages education and research, and recognizes the superior achievements of engineers. Dr. Charles M. Vest is president of the National Academy of Engineering.

The **Institute of Medicine** was established in 1970 by the National Academy of Sciences to secure the services of eminent members of appropriate professions in the examination of policy matters pertaining to the health of the public. The Institute acts under the responsibility given to the National Academy of Sciences by its congressional charter to be an adviser to the federal government and, upon its own initiative, to identify issues of medical care, research, and education. Dr. Harvey V. Fineberg is president of the Institute of Medicine.

The **National Research Council** was organized by the National Academy of Sciences in 1916 to associate the broad community of science and technology with the Academy's purposes of furthering knowledge and advising the federal government. Functioning in accordance with general policies determined by the Academy, the Council has become the principal operating agency of both the National Academy of Sciences and the National Academy of Engineering in providing services to the government, the public, and the scientific and engineering communities. The Council is administered jointly by both Academies and the Institute of Medicine. Dr. Ralph J. Cicerone and Dr. Charles M. Vest are chair and vice chair, respectively, of the National Research Council.

www.national-academies.org

v

Reviewers

This report has been reviewed in draft form by persons chosen for their diverse perspectives and technical expertise, in accordance with procedures approved by the National Research Council's (NRC's) Report Review Committee. The purpose of this independent review is to provide candid and critical comments that will assist the institution in making its published report as sound as possible and to ensure that the report meets institutional standards for objectivity, evidence, and responsiveness to the study charge. The review comments and draft manuscript remain confidential to protect the integrity of the deliberative process. We wish to thank the following individuals for their review of this report:

Scott Appleton, Ph.D., Altria Client Services, Inc.
John C. Bailar III, M.D., Ph.D., The University of Chicago
Robert Brook, M.D., University of Michigan Health System
Stanton A. Glantz, Ph.D., University of California, San Francisco School of Medicine
Christopher B. Granger, M.D., Duke University Medical Center
C. Arden Pope, M.S., Ph.D., Brigham Young University
Peter Rosen, M.D., Beth Israel Deaconess Medical Center
Jonathan M. Samet, M.D., M.S., Keck School of Medicine, University of Southern California
Michael Siegel, M.P.H., M.D., Boston University School of Medicine
Ponisseril Somasundaran, Ph.D., School of Engineering and Applied Science, Columbia University

Noel S. Weiss, M.D., Dr.P.H., School of Public Health and Community Medicine, University of Washington

Although the reviewers listed above have provided many constructive comments and suggestions, they were not asked to endorse the conclusions or recommendations nor did they see the final draft of the report before its release. The review of this report was overseen by **Floyd E. Bloom, M.D.,** The Scripps Research Institute, and **Rogene F. Henderson, Ph.D.,** Lovelace Respiratory Research Institute. Appointed by the NRC, they were responsible for making certain that an independent examination of this report was carried out in accordance with institutional procedures and that all review comments were carefully considered. Responsibility for the final content of this report rests entirely with the authoring committee and the institution.

Preface

The untimely death of a family member, friend, or coworker from acute cardiovascular events is a tragedy that repeats itself too many times each day. Overall age-adjusted mortality rates for heart disease have fallen significantly since the 1950s. Yet heart disease is still the leading cause of death in the United States. Ischemic heart disease killed nearly 424,900 people in the United States in 2006; or about half of the heart attacks that occurred that year.

Largely we have been focused on prevention of ischemic heart disease at the individual level, through identification of genetic risk factors and modification of lifestyle factors such as diet and physical fitness. Chief among these has been smoking and the role that it has played both in chronic and acute cardiac diseases.

More recently we have begun to appreciate that the environment plays a role. Years of careful research have elucidated a role for fine particulate air pollution formed from the combustion of fossil fuels in premature mortality due to cardiac disease. As smoking bans were put in place a number of researchers observed that there were reductions in hospital admissions and deaths due to acute cardiovascular events.

In carrying out our research it became clear that, while we have learned much about why and how tobacco smoke and particulate air pollution aggravate cardiovascular disease, there is still much to learn. The paucity of information about cardiovascular toxicity of chemicals, even those in tobacco smoke, is indicative of the lack of attention that has been paid to environmental contributions to cardiovascular disease.

It is hoped that our report will spur efforts to learn more. Too many people die prematurely each year to do otherwise.

I am deeply appreciative of the expert work of our committee members: Neal Benowitz, Aruni Bhatnagar, Francesca Dominici, Steve Fienberg, Gary Friedman, Kathie Hammond, Jiang He, Suzanne Oparil, Eric Peterson, and Ed Trapido. This was an extraordinary group who each provided important contributions to the final report. It has been a privilege and a pleasure to work with the Institute of Medicine staff, study director Michelle Catlin and her excellent team Rita Deng and Raina Sharma, as well as Jennifer Saunders and Naoko Ishibe, Sc.D. Without them, this report would not have been possible. I thank those who provided expert presentations and background materials and gave us much to think about: Captain Matthew McKenna, M.D., M.P.H. and Darwin Labarthe, M.D., M.P.H., Ph.D., Centers for Disease Control and Prevention; Stanton Glantz, Ph.D., University of California, San Francisco; Joel Kaufman, M.D., M.P.H., University of Washington, Seattle; Jon Samet, M.D., University of Southern California; Cynthia Hallett, American Nonsmokers' Rights Foundation; and Jared Jobe, Ph.D., National Heart, Lung and Blood Institute of the National Institutes of Health. In addition, I would like to thank individuals who assisted with the additional analyses of the committee: Aidan McDermott and Howard Chang, both from the Department of Biostatistics, Bloomberg School of Public Health, Johns Hopkins University. And, last, but certainly not least, I am appreciative of the time and effort offered by our reviewers, Floyd E. Bloom (monitor), Rogene F. Henderson (coordinator), Scott Appleton, John C. Bailar III, Robert Brook, Stanton A. Glantz, Christopher B. Granger, C. Arden Pope, Peter Rosen, Jonathan M. Samet, Michael Siegel, Ponisseril Somasundaran, and Noel S. Weiss.

> Lynn R. Goldman, *Chair*
> Committee on Secondhand Smoke Exposure and
> Acute Coronary Events

Contents

Summary

Secondhand smoke, also known as environmental tobacco smoke, is a complex mixture made up of particles and gases and includes smoke from burning cigarettes, cigars, and pipe tobacco (sidestream smoke) and exhaled mainstream smoke. This includes aged smoke that lingers after smoking ceases. Data suggest that exposure to secondhand smoke can result in heart disease in nonsmoking adults. Progress has been made recently in reducing involuntary exposure to secondhand smoke in workplaces, restaurants, and other public places in the United States and abroad, often through legislation that bans smoking. The effect of legislation to ban smoking in public places and workplaces on cardiovascular health of nonsmoking adults, however, remains a question.

CHARGE TO THE COMMITTEE

The Centers for Disease Control and Prevention (CDC) asked the Institute of Medicine (IOM) to convene an expert committee to assess the state of the science on the relationship between secondhand-smoke exposure and acute coronary events. This report addresses that charge. Specifically, the committee reviewed available scientific literature on secondhand-smoke exposure (including short-term exposure) and acute coronary events and characterized the state of the science on the topic with emphasis on the evidence of causality and knowledge gaps that future research should address. The committee was asked to address the following group of questions presented in Box S-1.

BOX S-1
Specific Questions to the Committee

The Centers for Disease Control and Prevention requested that the IOM convene an expert committee to assess the state of the science on the relationship between secondhand smoke exposure and acute coronary events. Specifically, the committee was to review available scientific literature on secondhand smoke exposure (including short-term exposure) and acute coronary events, and produce a report characterizing the state of the science on the topic, with emphasis on the evidence for causality and knowledge gaps that future research should address.

In conducting its work the committee was to address the following questions:

1. What is the current scientific consensus on the relationship between exposure to secondhand smoke and cardiovascular disease? What is the pathophysiology? What is the strength of the relationship?
2. Is there sufficient evidence to support the plausibility of a causal relation between secondhand smoke exposure and acute coronary events such as acute myocardial infarction and unstable angina? If yes, what is the pathophysiology? And what is the strength of the relationship?
3. Is it biologically plausible that a relatively brief (e.g., under 1 hour) secondhand smoke exposure incident could precipitate an acute

COMMITTEE'S APPROACH TO ITS CHARGE

In response to CDC's request, IOM convened an 11-member committee that included experts in secondhand-smoke exposure, the pharmacology and pathophysiology of secondhand smoke, clinical cardiology, epidemiology (including cardiovascular epidemiology), and statistics. The committee met three times, including two open information-gathering sessions at which the members heard from stakeholders and researchers, conducted an extensive literature search, and reviewed relevant publications. The committee reviewed both pathophysiologic and epidemiologic studies, and considered the findings of a 2006 report by the surgeon general of the U.S. Public Health Service, *The Health Consequences of Involuntary Exposure to Tobacco Smoke*.

Inherent in the committee's charge was the evaluation of three sets of relationships:

coronary event? If yes, what is known or suspected about how this risk may vary based upon absence or presence (and extent) of preexisting coronary artery disease?

4. What is the strength of the evidence for a causal relationship between indoor smoking bans and decreased risk of acute myocardial infarction?

5. What is a reasonable latency period between a decrease in secondhand smoke exposure and a decrease in risk of an acute myocardial infarction for an individual? What is a reasonable latency period between a decrease in population secondhand smoke exposure and a measurable decrease in acute myocardial infarction rates for a population?

6. What are the strengths and weaknesses of published population-based studies on the risk of acute myocardial infarction following the institution of comprehensive indoor smoking bans? In light of published studies' strengths and weaknesses, how much confidence is warranted in reported effect size estimates?

7. What factors would be expected to influence the effect size? For example, population age distribution, baseline level of secondhand smoke protection among nonsmokers, and level of secondhand smoke protection provided by the smoke-free law.

8. What are the most critical research gaps that should be addressed to improve our understanding of the impact of indoor air policies on acute coronary events? What studies should be performed to address these gaps?

1. the association between secondhand smoke exposure and cardiovascular disease, focusing on coronary heart disease and not stroke (Question 1);

2. the association between secondhand-smoke exposure and acute coronary events (Questions 2, 3, and 5); and

3. the association between smoking bans and acute coronary events (Questions 4, 5, 6, 7, and 8).

The committee reviewed the epidemiologic, clinical, and experimental studies relevant to the pathophysiology of secondhand smoke and cardiovascular effects, including coronary heart disease and acute coronary events. The pathophysiologic data not only provide insight into the potential modes of action underlying any effects of secondhand smoke on the cardiovascular system but also provide evidence on a causal relationship between secondhand-smoke exposure and adverse cardiovascular outcomes.

Eleven publications played a key role in the committee's evaluation of smoking bans and were a focus of the committee's deliberations. Those publications assessed the effects of smoking bans on acute coronary events in the following locations: three on overlapping regions of Italy after implementation of a national smoking ban; two on the effects of a smoking ban in the city of Pueblo, Colorado, one with 18 months and one with 3 years of followup; and one each on the effects of smoking bans in Helena, Montana; Monroe County, Indiana; Bowling Green, Ohio; New York state; Saskatoon, Canada; and Scotland. Those 11 studies are observational studies that examined changes in heart-attack rates after implementation of smoking bans, and they were not designed to answer questions about all three of the associations listed above. Most of them did not measure individual exposures to secondhand smoke or the smoking status of individuals; they were designed to evaluate the association between smoking bans and heart attacks, not the effects of secondhand-smoke exposure. The studies of the smoking bans in Monroe County, Indiana, and Scotland, however, had data on smoking status and conducted analyses only in nonsmokers. Those two studies were designed to assess the association between secondhand-smoke exposure and heart attacks.

SECONDHAND-SMOKE EXPOSURE AND CORONARY HEART DISEASE

The results of both case–control and cohort studies carried out in multiple populations consistently indicate that exposure to secondhand smoke increases the risk of coronary heart disease by about 25–30%, with higher estimates in the few studies that had better quantitative assessment of exposure. Data from epidemiologic studies with quantitative exposure assessment and from animal studies demonstrate a dose–response relationship. The epidemiologic evidence indicates increased risks even at the lowest exposures and a steep initial rise in risk followed by a gradual increase with increasing exposure. The pathophysiology of coronary heart disease and results of human chamber studies and laboratory studies of the constituents of secondhand smoke make such a relationship biologically plausible. The pathophysiology through which cigarette-smoking and exposure to secondhand smoke induce cardiovascular disease is complex and probably involves multiple chemical agents inasmuch as secondhand smoke itself and a number of its components have been shown to exert chronic cardiovascular toxicity. The association is also consistent with known associations between particulate matter (PM), a major constituent of secondhand smoke, and coronary heart disease.

On the basis of its review of the data, the committee concurs with the current scientific consensus in the 2006 surgeon general's report that "the evidence is sufficient to infer a causal relationship between exposure to secondhand smoke and increased risks of coronary heart disease morbidity and mortality among both men and women." Although the committee found strong evidence of an association between chronic secondhand-smoke exposure and coronary heart disease and the relative risks are consistent, the evidence that might be used to determine the magnitude of the association—that is, the number of cases of disease that are attributable to secondhand-smoke exposure—is not as strong. Furthermore, many other individual lifestyle, community, and societal factors that lead to coronary heart disease could influence the magnitude of the effect in studies. The committee therefore did not estimate the size of the effect or the attributable risk.

SECONDHAND-SMOKE EXPOSURE AND
ACUTE CORONARY EVENTS

Two of the epidemiologic studies reviewed by the committee analyzed changes in the hospitalization rate for acute coronary events after the implementation of smoking bans. They reported only events in nonsmokers (Monroe, Indiana) or analyzed nonsmokers and smokers separately (Scotland). Those studies provided direct evidence related to secondhand-smoke exposure and acute coronary events. Both studies showed reductions in the relative risk of acute coronary events in nonsmokers with the decrease in secondhand-smoke exposure that occurred after implementation of smoking bans. Because of differences between the studies (for example, in population and population size and in analysis), they did not provide sufficient evidence of the magnitude of the decrease in relative risk. The effect seen after implementation of smoking bans is consistent with data from the INTERHEART study, a case–control study of 15,152 first cases of acute myocardial infarction (MI, or heart attack) in 262 centers in 52 countries. Exposure to secondhand smoke increased the risk of nonfatal acute MI in a graded manner, with adjusted odds ratios of 1.24 (95% confidence interval [CI], 1.17–1.32) and 1.62 (95% CI, 1.45–1.81) in those least exposed (1–7 hours of exposure per week) and those most exposed (at least 22 hours of exposure per week), respectively. In contrast, a study that used data from the Western New York Health Study collected from 1995 to 2001 found that secondhand-smoke exposure was not significantly associated with an increase in the risk of MI. That study, however, looked at lifetime cumulative exposure to secondhand smoke, which is a different exposure metric from what was used in the other studies and does not take into account how recent the exposure was.

The nine other key epidemiologic studies that looked at smoking bans provided indirect evidence of an association between secondhand-smoke exposure and acute coronary events. It is not possible to separate the effect of smoking bans in reducing exposure to secondhand smoke from their effect in reducing active smoking in those studies, because they did not have individual smoking status or secondhand-smoke exposure concentrations; however, monitoring studies of airborne tracers[1] and biomarkers[2] of exposure to secondhand smoke have demonstrated that exposure to secondhand smoke is dramatically reduced after the implementation of smoking bans. Thus, those studies provided indirect evidence that at least part of the decrease in acute coronary events seen after implementation of smoking bans could be mediated by a decrease in exposure to secondhand smoke. It is not possible to determine the magnitude of the effect that is attributable to changes in nonsmokers compared with smokers. It should also be noted that although the studies have limitations related to their taking advantage of natural experiments, they did directly evaluate the effects of an intervention (smoking bans and concomitant activities) on a health outcome of interest (acute coronary events).

As in the case of longer-term cardiovascular effects, experimental data have demonstrated that an association between secondhand-smoke exposure and acute coronary events is biologically plausible. Experimental studies in humans, animals, and cell cultures have demonstrated short-term effects of secondhand smoke, its components (such as oxidants, PM, acrolein, polycyclic aromatic hydrocarbons, benzene, and metals), or both on the cardiovascular system. There is sufficient evidence from such studies to infer that acute exposure to secondhand smoke at concentrations relevant to population exposures induces endothelial dysfunction, increases thrombosis, and potentially affects plaque stability adversely. Those effects occur at magnitudes relevant to the pathogenesis of acute coronary events. Furthermore, indirect evidence obtained from studies of ambient PM supports the notion that exposure to the PM in secondhand smoke could trigger acute coronary events or induce arrhythymogenesis in vulnerable myocardium.

None of the studies had information on the duration or pattern of exposure of individuals to secondhand smoke. That is, there was no information on how long or how often individuals were exposed before or after implementation of smoking bans. For example, it is not known whether individuals were exposed to high concentrations sporadically for short periods, to low concentrations more consistently, or both. Without that infor-

---

[1] Airborne measures of exposure, such as the unique tracer nicotine or the less specific tracer PM, can demonstrate the contribution of different sources or venues of an exposure but do not reflect the true dose.

[2] Biomarkers of exposure to tobacco smoke, such as serum and salivary cotinine concentrations, integrate all sources of exposure and inhalation rates, but because of a short half-life, they reflect only recent exposures.

mation, the committee could not determine whether acute exposures were triggering acute coronary events, chronic exposures were causing chronic damage that eventually resulted in acute coronary events, or a combination of chronic damage and an acute-exposure trigger led to the increased risk of acute coronary events.

The combination of the evidence from the epidemiologic studies and the information from the experimental studies and studies of PM is sufficient to support an inference of a causal relationship between exposure to secondhand smoke and acute coronary events. Although data from experimental studies have indicated that cardiovascular effects are seen after very brief exposures (less than 1 hour), the data from most of the epidemiologic studies do not include the duration of exposures before smoking bans, so the committee could not estimate the length of exposure required to increase the risk of acute MI.

SMOKING BANS AND ACUTE CORONARY EVENTS

All 11 key epidemiologic studies are relevant and informative with respect to the questions posed to the committee, and overall they support an association between smoking bans and a decrease in the incidence of acute coronary events. They show remarkable consistency: all the studies showed decreases in the rate of heart attacks (acute MIs) after implementation of smoking bans. The decreases ranged from about 6 to 47%, depending on the study and the form of analysis. The consistency in the direction of change gave the committee confidence that smoking bans decrease the rate of heart attacks. It is important to note that contextual factors associated with a ban—such as public comment periods, information announcing the ban, notices about the impending changes, education and outreach efforts on the adverse health effects of secondhand smoke, and support for smoking-cessation programs—are difficult, if not impossible, to separate from the impact of the ban itself and could vary from ban to ban. Therefore, committee conclusions regarding the effects of bans refer to the combined effects of different types of legislation and those contextual factors.

The committee was unable to determine the magnitude of effect on the basis of the 11 studies, because of variability among and uncertainties within them. Characteristics of smoking bans vary greatly among the locations studied and must be taken into account in reviewing results of epidemiologic studies. Those characteristics include the venues covered by the bans (such as offices, other workplaces, restaurants, and bars) and compliance with and enforcement of the bans. Other differences or potential differences among the studies include the length of followup after implementation, population characteristics (such as underlying rates of acute coronary events and prevalence of other risk factors for acute coronary events, including diabetes and obesity) and size, secondhand-smoke exposure levels before and after implementation, preexisting smoking bans or restrictions, smoking rates, and method of statistical analysis. The time between implementation of a ban and decreases in secondhand smoke and acute cardiovascular events cannot be determined from the studies, because of the variability among the studies and indeed the difficulty of determining the precise time of onset of a ban. On the basis of its review of the available experimental and epidemiologic literature, including relevant literature on air pollution and PM, the committee concludes that there is a causal relationship between smoking bans and decreases in acute coronary events.

RESPONSES TO SPECIFIC QUESTIONS TO THE COMMITTEE

The committee was tasked with responding to a number of specific questions. The questions and the committee's responses are presented below.

1. *What is the current scientific consensus on the relationship between exposure to secondhand smoke and cardiovascular disease? What is the pathophysiology? What is the strength of the relationship?*

On the basis of the available studies of chronic exposure to secondhand smoke and cardiovascular disease, the committee concludes that there is scientific consensus that there is a causal relationship between secondhand-smoke exposure and cardiovascular disease. The results of a number of meta-analyses of the epidemiologic studies showed increases of 25–30% in the risk of cardiovascular disease caused by various exposures. The studies include some that use serum cotinine concentration as a biomarker of exposure and show a dose–response relationship. The pathophysiologic data are consistent with that relationship, as are the data from studies of air pollution and PM. The data in support of the relationship are consistent, but the committee could not calculate a point estimate of the magnitude of the effect (that is, the effect size) given the variable strength of the relationship, differences among studies, poor assessment of secondhand-smoke exposure, and variation in concomitant underlying risk factors.

2. *Is there sufficient evidence to support the plausibility of a causal relation between secondhand smoke exposure and acute coronary events such as acute myocardial infarction and unstable angina? If yes, what is the pathophysiology? And what is the strength of the relationship?*

The evidence reviewed by the committee is consistent with a causal relationship between secondhand-smoke exposure and acute coronary events, such as acute MI. It is unknown whether acute exposure, chronic exposure, or a combination of the two underlies the occurrence of acute coronary events, inasmuch as the duration or pattern of exposure in individuals is not known. The evidence includes the results of two key studies that have information on individual smoking status and that showed decreases in risks of acute coronary events in nonsmokers after implementation of a smoking ban. Those studies are supported by information from other smoking-ban studies (although these do not have information on individual smoking status, other exposure-assessment studies have demonstrated that secondhand-smoke exposure decreases after implementation of a smoking ban) and by the large body of literature on PM, especially $PM_{2.5}$, a constituent of secondhand smoke. The evidence is not yet comprehensive enough to determine a detailed mode of action for the relationship between secondhand-smoke exposure and a variety of intervening and preexisting conditions in predisposing to cardiac events. However, experimental studies have shown effects that are consistent with pathogenic factors in acute coronary events. Although the committee has confidence in the evidence of an association between chronic secondhand-smoke exposure and acute coronary events, the evidence on the magnitude of the association is less convincing, so the committee did not estimate that magnitude (that is, the effect size).

3. *Is it biologically plausible that a relatively brief (e.g., under 1 hour) secondhand smoke exposure incident could precipitate an acute coronary event? If yes, what is known or suspected about how this risk may vary based upon absence or presence (and extent) of preexisting coronary artery disease?*

There is no direct evidence that a relatively brief exposure to secondhand smoke can precipitate an acute coronary event; few published studies have addressed that question. The circumstantial evidence of such a relationship, however, is compelling. The strongest evidence comes from air-pollution research, especially research on PM. Although the source of the PM can affect its toxicity, particle size in secondhand smoke is comparable with that in air pollution, and research has demonstrated a similarity between cardiovascular effects of PM and of secondhand smoke. Some studies have demonstrated rapid effects of brief secondhand-smoke exposure (for example, on platelet aggregation and endothelial function), but more research is necessary to delineate how secondhand smoke produces cardiovascular effects and the role of underlying preexisting coronary arterial disease in determining susceptibility to the effects. Given the data on PM, especially those from time-series studies, which indicate that a relatively brief exposure can precipitate an acute coronary event, and the fact that

PM is a major component of secondhand smoke, the committee concludes that it is biologically plausible for a relatively brief exposure to secondhand smoke to precipitate an acute coronary event.

With respect to how the risk might vary in the presence or absence of preexisting coronary arterial disease, it is generally assumed that acute coronary events are more likely to occur in people who have some level of preexisting disease, although that underlying disease is often subclinical. There are not enough data on the presence of preexisting coronary arterial disease in the populations studied to assess the extent to which the absence or presence of such preexisting disease affects the cardiovascular risk posed by secondhand-smoke exposure.

    4.   *What is the strength of the evidence for a causal relationship between indoor smoking bans and decreased risk of acute myocardial infarction?*

The key intervention studies that have evaluated the effects of indoor smoking bans consistently have shown a decreased risk of heart attack. Research has also indicated that secondhand-smoke exposure is causally related to heart attacks, that smoking bans decrease secondhand-smoke exposure, and that a relationship between secondhand-smoke exposure and acute coronary events is biologically plausible. All the relevant studies have shown an association in a direction consistent with a causal relationship (although the committee was unable to estimate the magnitude of the association), and the committee therefore concludes that the evidence is sufficient to infer a causal relationship.

    5.   *What is a reasonable latency period between a decrease in secondhand smoke exposure and a decrease in risk of an acute myocardial infarction for an individual? What is a reasonable latency period between a decrease in population secondhand smoke exposure and a measurable decrease in acute myocardial infarction rates for a population?*

No direct information is available on the time between a decrease in secondhand-smoke exposure and a decrease in the risk of a heart attack in an individual. Data on PM, however, have shown effects on the heart within 24 hours, and this supports a period of less than 24 hours. At the population level, results of the key intervention studies reviewed by the committee are for the most part consistent with a decrease in risk as early as a month following reductions in secondhand-smoke exposure; however, given the variability in the studies and the lack of data on the precise timing of interventions, the smoking-ban studies do not provide adequate information on the time it takes to see decreases in heart attacks.

6. *What are the strengths and weaknesses of published population-based studies on the risk of acute myocardial infarction following the institution of comprehensive indoor smoking bans? In light of published studies' strengths and weaknesses, how much confidence is warranted in reported effect size estimates?*

Some of the weaknesses of the published population-based studies of the risk of MI after implementation of smoking bans are

- Limitations associated with an open study population and, in some cases, with the use of a small sample.
- Concurrent interventions that reduce the observed effect of a smoking ban.
- Lack of exposure-assessment criteria and measurements.
- Lack of information collected on the time between the cessation of exposure to secondhand smoke and changes in disease rates.
- Differences between control and intervention groups.
- Nonexperimental design of studies (by necessity).
- Lack of assessment of the sensitivity of results to the assumptions made in the statistical analysis.

The different studies had different strengths and weaknesses in relation to the assessment of the effects of smoking bans. For example, the Scottish study had such strengths as prospective design and serum cotinine measurements. The Saskatoon study had the advantage of comprehensive hospital records, and the Monroe County study excluded smokers. The population-based studies of the risk of heart attack after the institution of comprehensive smoking bans were consistent in showing an association between the smoking bans and a decrease in the risk of acute coronary events, and this strengthened the committee's confidence in the existence of the association. However, because of the weaknesses discussed above and the variability among the studies, the committee has little confidence in the magnitude of the effects and, therefore, thought it inappropriate to attempt to estimate an effect size from such disparate designs and measures.

7. *What factors would be expected to influence the effect size? For example, population age distribution, baseline level of secondhand smoke protection among nonsmokers, and level of secondhand smoke protection provided by the smoke-free law.*

A number of factors that vary among the key studies can influence effect size. Although some of the studies found different effects in different age groups, these were not consistently identified. One major factor is the size of the difference in secondhand-smoke exposure before and after implementation of a ban, which would vary and depends on: the magnitude of exposure before the ban, which is influenced by the baseline level of smoking and preexisting smoking bans or restrictions; and the magnitude of exposure after implementation of the ban, which is influenced by the extent of the ban, enforcement of and compliance with the ban, changes in social norms of smoking behaviors, and remaining exposure in areas not covered by the ban (for example, in private vehicles and homes). The baseline rate of acute coronary events or cardiovascular disease could influence the effect size, as would the prevalence of other risk factors for acute coronary events, such as obesity, diabetes, and age.

8. *What are the most critical research gaps that should be addressed to improve our understanding of the impact of indoor air policies on acute coronary events? What studies should be performed to address these gaps?*

The committee identified the following gaps and research needs as those most critical for improving understanding of the effect of indoor-air policies on acute coronary events:

- The committee found a relative paucity of data on environmental cardiotoxicity of secondhand smoke compared with other disease end points related to secondhand smoke, such as carcinogenicity and reproductive toxicity. Research should develop standard definitions of cardiotoxic end points in pathophysiologic studies (for example, specific results on standard assays) and a classification system for cardiotoxic agents (similar to the International Agency for Research on Cancer classification of carcinogens). Established cardiotoxicity assays for environmental exposures and consistent definitions of adverse outcomes of such tests would improve investigations of the cardiotoxicity of secondhand smoke and its components and identify potential end points for the investigation of the effects of indoor-air policies on acute coronary events.
- The committee found a lack of a system for surveillance of the prevalence of cardiovascular disease and of the incidence of acute coronary events in the United States. Surveillance of incidence and prevalence trends would allow secular trends to be taken into account better and to be compared among different populations to

establish the effects of indoor-air policies. Although some national databases and surveys include cardiovascular end points, a national database that tracks hospital admission rates and deaths from acute coronary events, similar to the SEER database for cancer, would improve epidemiologic studies.

- The committee found a lack of understanding of a mechanism that leads to plaque rupture and from that to an acute coronary event and of how secondhand smoke affects that process. Additional research is necessary to develop reliable biomarkers of early effects on plaque vulnerability to rupture and to improve the design of pathophysiologic studies of secondhand smoke that examine effects of exposure on plaque stability.

- All 11 key studies reviewed by the committee have strengths and limitations due to their study design, and none was designed to test the hypothesis that secondhand-smoke exposure causes cardiovascular disease or acute coronary events. Because of those limitations and the consequent variability in results, the committee did not have enough information to estimate the magnitude of the decrease in cardiovascular risk due to smoking bans or to a decrease in secondhand-smoke exposure. A large, well-designed study could permit estimation of the magnitude of the effect. An ideal study would be prospective; would have individual-level data on smoking status; would account for potential confounders, including other risk factors for cardiovascular events (such as obesity and age), would have biomarkers of mainstream and secondhand-smoke exposures (such as blood cotinine concentrations); and would have enough cases to allow separate analyses of smokers and nonsmokers or, ideally, stratification of cases by cotinine concentrations to examine the dose–response relationship. Such a study could be specifically designed for secondhand smoke or potentially could take advantage of existing cohort studies that might have data available or attainable for investigating secondhand-smoke exposure and its cardiovascular effects, such as was done with the INTERHEART study. Existing studies that could be explored to determine their utility and applicability to questions related to secondhand smoke include the Multi-Ethnic Study of Atherosclerosis (MESA) study, the American Cancer Society's CPS-3, the European Prospective Investigation of Cancer (EPIC), the Framingham Heart Study, and the Jackson Heart Study. Researchers should clearly articulate the assumptions used in their statistical models and include analysis of the sensitivity of results to model choice and assumptions.

1

Introduction

Secondhand smoke, also known as environmental tobacco smoke, is a complex mixture of gases and particles and includes smoke from burning cigarettes, cigars, and pipe tobacco (sidestream smoke) and exhaled mainstream smoke (Cal EPA, 2005a; HHS, 2005). According to the National Toxicology Program, sidestream smoke and mainstream smoke contain "at least 250 chemicals known to be toxic or carcinogenic" (HHS, 2005). Exposure to secondhand smoke results in heart disease, lung cancer, and other diseases in nonsmoking adults (Cal EPA, 2005a; HHS, 2005). Although much research has focused on the carcinogenic properties of smoke, this report focuses on its cardiovascular effects.

In 1972, the U.S. Office of the Surgeon General released its first statement on the public-health hazard to people suffering from coronary heart disease posed by secondhand smoke in *The Health Consequences of Smoking* (HHS, 1972). In 1986, it emphasized the need for further examination of the relationship between "involuntary smoking" and cardiovascular disease in *The Health Consequences of Involuntary Smoking* (HHS, 1986). Most recently, in *The Health Consequences of Involuntary Exposure to Tobacco Smoke* (HHS, 2006), it concluded that exposure to secondhand smoke could have immediate adverse effects on the cardiovascular system in adults and that it causes coronary heart disease.

Smoking cessation has been associated with reduced risk of coronary heart disease. The speed and magnitude of risk reduction after smoking cessation, however, have been debated (Critchley and Capewell, 2003; Dobson et al., 1991; Doll and Peto, 1976; Gordon et al., 1974; Negri et al., 1994). Some studies found that risk could decline to that of a lifelong nonsmoker

(Dobson et al., 1991; Gordon et al., 1974; Lightwood and Glantz, 1997), and others have suggested that some residual excess risk remains (Negri et al., 1994; Teo et al., 2006). Studies have reported a range of latency periods for such risk reduction, with the shortest being 2 or 3 years (Gordon et al., 1974). In addition, the 1990 report *The Health Benefits of Smoking Cessation: A Report of the Surgeon General* (HHS, 1990) and the National Cancer Institute's *Monograph 8: Changes in Cigarette-Related Disease Risks and Their Implications for Prevention and Control* (NCI, 1997) discussed the cardiovascular benefits of smoking cessation. On the basis of a systematic review of 20 cohort studies, Critchley and Capewell (2003) estimated that there was a 36% reduction in mortality in patients with coronary heart disease who quit smoking compared with those who continued smoking. Their data provide evidence that limitation of secondhand-smoke exposure should reduce risk of mortality from coronary heart disease substantially.

The high prevalence of secondhand smoke and consequently the increased risk of coronary heart disease in the U.S. general population have important implications for public health. According to the Third National Health and Nutrition Examination Survey (NHANES III), about 43% of nonsmoking children and 37% of nonsmoking adults are exposed to secondhand smoke in the United States (Pirkle et al., 1996). The California Environmental Protection Agency has estimated that 46,000 (range, 22,700–69,600) excess cardiac deaths in the United States each year are attributable to secondhand-smoke exposure at home and in the workplace (Cal EPA, 2005b). Thus, home and workplace exposure can potentially produce a substantial burden of avoidable deaths from coronary heart disease. Similarly, Lightwood et al. (2009) recently estimated that at the 1999 to 2004 levels, passive smoking leads to 21,800 to 75,100 deaths from coronary heart disease and 38,100 to 128,900 myocardial infarctions annually.

Progress has been made recently in reducing involuntary exposure to secondhand smoke in workplaces, restaurants, and other public places in the United States and abroad. According to the surgeon general's 2006 report (HHS, 2006), the percentage of U.S. nonsmokers 4 years old and older who are exposed to secondhand smoke decreased from 88% in 1988–1991 to 43% in 2001–2002, improving on the Healthy People 2010 target of 45% (HHS, 2000). Despite the improvement, some 126 million nonsmokers living in the United States in 2000 were still being exposed to secondhand smoke. Data reviewed in the surgeon general's 2006 report indicate that smoke-free policies are the most economical and effective way to reduce secondhand-smoke exposure (HHS, 2006); the effect of legislation to ban smoking in public places and workplaces on cardiovascular health of nonsmoking adults, however, remains a question.

CHARGE TO THE COMMITTEE

The Centers for Disease Control and Prevention (CDC) asked the Institute of Medicine (IOM) to convene an expert committee to assess the state of the science on the relationship between secondhand-smoke exposure and acute coronary events. This report addresses that charge. Specifically, the committee reviewed available scientific literature on secondhand-smoke exposure (including short-term exposure) and acute coronary events, with emphasis on evidence of causality and on knowledge gaps that future research should address. To accomplish its task, the committee was asked to address a series of specific questions, which are presented in Box 1-1.

COMMITTEE'S APPROACH TO ITS CHARGE

Inherent in that charge is the evaluation for the following three sets of relationships:

1. the association between secondhand smoke exposure and cardiovascular disease, focusing on coronary heart disease and not stroke (Question 1);
2. the association between secondhand smoke exposure and acute coronary events (Questions 2, 3, and 5); and
3. the association between smoking bans and acute coronary events (Questions 4, 5, 6, 7, and 8).

In response to CDC's request, IOM convened an 11-member committee to assess the state of the science on the relationship between secondhand-smoke exposure and acute coronary events. The committee included experts in secondhand-smoke exposure, the pharmacology and pathophysiology of secondhand smoke, clinical cardiology, epidemiology (including cardiovascular epidemiology), and statistics. The committee met three times, including two open information-gathering sessions at which the members heard from stakeholders and researchers. The appendix presents the agendas of the public meetings.

The committee also conducted an extensive literature search and reviewed relevant publications. To ensure that it was aware of all relevant studies, the committee searched medical-literature databases from 1997 to the present with keywords that included *tobacco smoke pollution, secondhand smoke, passive smoking, smoke-free, smoking bans, and smoking ordinance*. The databases searched include EMBASE, MedLine, CRISP, Clinical Trials.gov, the New York Academy of Sciences GreyLit, NACCHO, and WorldCat. Databases were searched for seasonal changes and long-term trends in acute coronary events before and after smoking-ban legislation,

---

BOX 1-1
Specific Questions to the Committee

The Centers for Disease Control and Prevention requested that the IOM convene an expert committee to assess the state of the science on the relationship between secondhand smoke exposure and acute coronary events. Specifically, the committee was to review available scientific literature on secondhand smoke exposure (including short-term exposure) and acute coronary events, and produce a report characterizing the state of the science on the topic, with emphasis on the evidence for causality and knowledge gaps that future research should address.

In conducting its work the committee was to address the following questions:

1. What is the current scientific consensus on the relationship between exposure to secondhand smoke and cardiovascular disease? What is the pathophysiology? What is the strength of the relationship?
2. Is there sufficient evidence to support the plausibility of a causal relation between secondhand smoke exposure and acute coronary events such as acute myocardial infarction and unstable angina? If yes, what is the pathophysiology? And what is the strength of the relationship?
3. Is it biologically plausible that a relatively brief (e.g., under 1 hour) secondhand smoke exposure incident could precipitate an acute

---

for exposure data, and for data on pathophysiologic effects of second-hand smoke that could underlie any acute coronary events that might be seen. The literature searches identified thousands of publications relevant to secondhand-smoke pathophysiology and health effects and relevant to smoking bans, from which the committee identified studies to be discussed in this report.

The committee focused on the pathophysiologic, exposure, and epidemiologic studies that it thought most pertinent to its charge, including studies that looked at the cardiotoxic components of secondhand smoke (such as particulate matter). The committee evaluated in great detail 11 publications that specifically assessed the effect of smoking bans on the incidence of acute coronary events (see Chapter 5). Those publications looked at the effects of eight smoking bans in different locations: three publications on overlapping regions of Italy after implementation of a national smoking ban (Barone-Adesi et al., 2006; Cesaroni et al., 2008; Vasselli et al., 2008);

coronary event? If yes, what is known or suspected about how this risk may vary based upon absence or presence (and extent) of preexisting coronary artery disease?

4. What is the strength of the evidence for a causal relationship between indoor smoking bans and decreased risk of acute myocardial infarction?

5. What is a reasonable latency period between a decrease in secondhand smoke exposure and a decrease in risk of an acute myocardial infarction for an individual? What is a reasonable latency period between a decrease in population secondhand smoke exposure and a measurable decrease in acute myocardial infarction rates for a population?

6. What are the strengths and weaknesses of published population-based studies on the risk of acute myocardial infarction following the institution of comprehensive indoor smoking bans? In light of published studies' strengths and weaknesses, how much confidence is warranted in reported effect size estimates?

7. What factors would be expected to influence the effect size? For example, population age distribution, baseline level of secondhand smoke protection among nonsmokers, and level of secondhand smoke protection provided by the smoke-free law.

8. What are the most critical research gaps that should be addressed to improve our understanding of the impact of indoor air policies on acute coronary events? What studies should be performed to address these gaps?

two publications on the effects of a smoking ban in Pueblo, Colorado—one with 18 months of data (Bartecchi et al., 2006) and one with 3 years of data (CDC, 2009); and one publication each on the effects of smoking bans in Helena, Montana (Sargent et al., 2004), Monroe County, Indiana (Seo and Torabi, 2007), Bowling Green, Ohio (Khuder et al., 2007), New York state (Juster et al., 2007), Saskatoon, Canada (Lemstra et al., 2008), and Scotland (Pell et al., 2008). Those 11 publications, which are observational studies examining changes in heart-attack rates following the implementation of a smoking ban, are not designed to answer questions regarding all three of the associations discussed previously. Most of the studies do not measure individual exposures to secondhand smoke or the smoking status of individuals. Those studies, therefore, are designed to evaluate the association between smoking bans and heart attacks, not the effects of secondhand smoke exposure. The publications on the smoking bans in Monroe County, Indiana (Seo and Torabi, 2007), and Scotland (Pell et al., 2008), however, have data on smoking status and have conducted analyses only in nonsmokers. Those two studies, therefore, are designed to assess the association between secondhand smoke exposure and heart attacks.

For the purpose of addressing its charge, the committee defined *secondhand smoke* as a complex mixture that is made up of gases and particles and includes smoke from burning cigarettes, cigars, and pipe tobacco (sidestream smoke) and exhaled mainstream smoke. This includes aged smoke that lingers after smoking ceases. In consultation with CDC, the committee interpreted the charge to focus on coronary heart disease, not stroke, and mainly on the association of secondhand smoke with acute coronary events. Most of the 11 key publications, and the present report, examined in this report defined *acute coronary events* as acute myocardial infarction, including both "ST elevation myocardial infarction" (STEMI) and "non-ST elevation myocardial infarction" (NSTEMI). Other studies included unstable angina (new-onset, accelerating, and rest angina) and sudden cardiac death. The American Heart Association (AHA) defines *sudden cardiac death* as death resulting from an abrupt loss of heart function (AHA, 2009). *Acute coronary syndrome* is an umbrella term used to describe any group of clinical symptoms compatible with acute myocardial ischemia, which includes those cardiac events (AHA, 2009). The codes associated with acute coronary syndrome in the ninth revision of *International Classification of Diseases* include 410.xx for acute myocardial infarction and 411.xx for other acute and sub-acute forms of ischemic heart disease. *Chronic cardiovascular disease* (chronic CVD) refers to diseases that involve the cardiovascular system, including the heart and circulation, and are longer- term conditions relative to an acute event, such as a heart attack. Chronic CVD increases the risk of a cardiovascular event.

The committee differentiates between smoking bans and smoking restrictions and between smokers and nonsmokers. The definitions that the committee uses in this report for those and other terms are presented in Box 1-2.

In response to specific questions in the committee's charge (see Box 1-1), the committee also reviewed the scientific evidence and current scientific consensus on the association between secondhand-smoke exposure and cardiovascular disease in general (Question 1) and the evidence related to the biologic plausibility of a causal association between secondhand-smoke exposure and acute coronary events (Question 2). Data on cardiovascular disease and data on acute coronary events are presented in Chapter 2. Because secondhand smoke and air pollution contain many of the same constituents (such as particulate matter), the committee also discussed the association between exposure to some constituents of air pollution and acute coronary

---

BOX 1-2
Definitions

Smoker. A person that smokes tobacco products.

Nonsmoker. A person that does not smoke tobacco products.

Secondhand smoke: A complex mixture that is made up of gases and particles and includes smoke from burning cigarettes, cigars, and pipe tobacco (sidestream smoke) and exhaled mainstream smoke. This includes aged smoke that lingers after smoking ceases.

Acute coronary event: Acute myocardial infarction, including both "ST elevation myocardial infarction" (STEMI) and "non-ST elevation myocardial infarction" (NSTEMI).

Smoking ban: A legal mandate that prohibits use of lit tobacco products in designated public or private places (such as office buildings).

Smoking restriction: A legal mandate that limits the use of lit tobacco products to specified areas in designated public or private places (such as office buildings).

---

events. The committee presents information on air pollutants in this report relevant to the biologic plausibility of associations between secondhand smoke and cardiovascular disease, but it did not conduct an extensive literature review on the topic of air-pollutant health effects.

SOURCES OF UNCERTAINTY IN KEY STUDIES

As discussed above, 11 publications report studies of the effect of smoking bans on the incidence of acute coronary events. The design of those studies created challenges to their interpretation and uncertainties in their conclusions. Those challenges include: the lack of a closed study population, the need to disentangle the effects of the smoking ban itself from other concurrent activities that could affect smoking behaviors, exposure assessment, the time between cessation of exposure and changes in disease rates, the use of less-than-perfect control groups, the question of the biologic plausibility of the effect, the necessarily nonexperimental nature of the studies, the need to clarify hypotheses and variability in statistical analyses.[1] The challenges are discussed in detail in later chapters in this report; they are summarized briefly below.

Ideally, when evaluating an effect in a population that population would be closed, that is, it does not change with time (for example, in a clinical trial). The studies that examined the effect of smoking bans were inevitably not closed populations; people were free to move back and forth between areas with and without bans. The committee discusses the potential impact of that migration on the results of the studies in Chapter 7, but generally it would be expected to attenuate the estimated effects of smoking bans in studies unless smokers were selectively moving out of areas with bans and into areas without bans.

In examining the effect of any population intervention, ideally there is a defined time at which the intervention is implemented so that the reduction in adverse outcomes attributable to the intervention can be estimated, and that other interventions that could affect the outcome being studied can be accounted for. In this case, the intervention—the implementation of a smoking ban—does not necessarily occur at a precise time given that voluntary bans or other smoking restrictions may already be in place for a subset of the study population when the ban is imposed. Moreover, bans may vary in scope, enforcement may differ among areas and vary over time, and a smoking ban is often (but not necessarily) accompanied by other interventions, such as smoking-cessation and education efforts (see Figure 1-1). When the committee draws conclusions regarding the effects of smoking bans, therefore, it cannot completely distinguish the effects of bans from the effects of policies and activities that are occurring concurrently. At a minimum, the process leading to adoption of a ban is likely to generate awareness about smoking-related risks. These issues surrounding smoking bans are discussed further in Chapter 7, which also discusses how they might have affected the 11 key publications.

Three issues are important in assessing exposure. First, although two of the 11 studies have information on smoking statues, the other studies do not have the data available to determine the smoking status of people who have acute coronary events. Smokers might quit or decrease their smoking in anticipation of or after a ban is implemented (IOM, 2007). If a study does not look only at nonsmokers or does not determine the smoking status of people who have acute coronary events, it cannot separate decreases in acute coronary events in nonsmokers that are due to lowering of secondhand-smoke exposure from decreases that are due to smoking

---

[1] Dr. J. Kaufman presented to the committee at its January 30, 2009, meeting. The committee found the framework of that presentation useful for organizing its comments on the key studies.

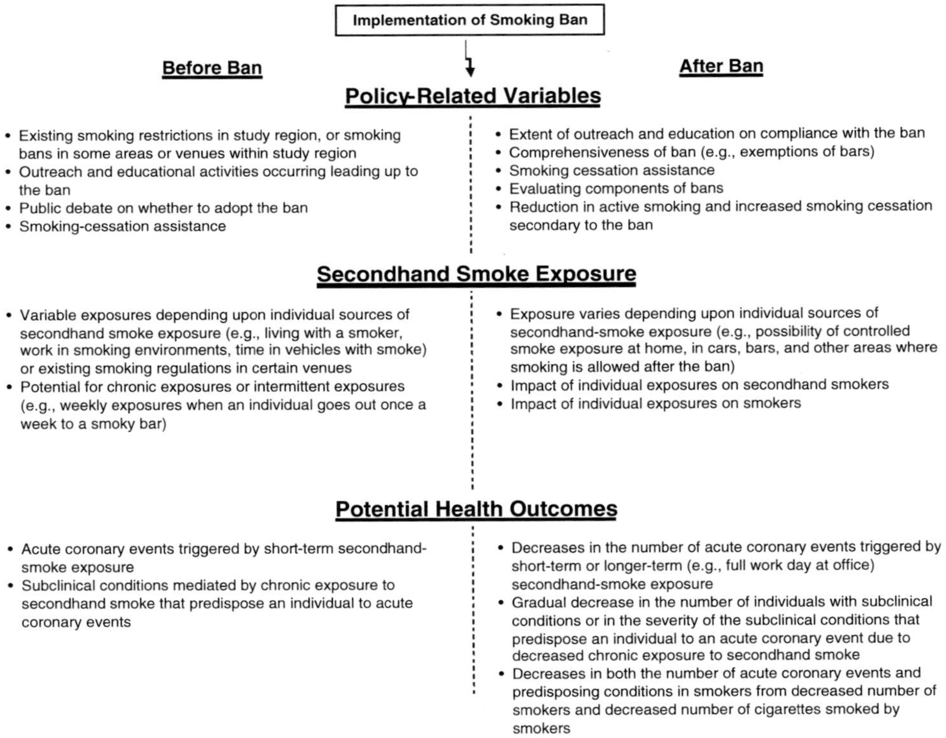

Implementation of Smoking Ban

Before Ban

After Ban

Policy-Related Variables

Before Ban:
- Existing smoking restrictions in study region, or smoking bans in some areas or venues within study region
- Outreach and educational activities occurring leading up to the ban
- Public debate on whether to adopt the ban
- Smoking-cessation assistance

After Ban:
- Extent of outreach and education on compliance with the ban
- Comprehensiveness of ban (e.g., exemptions of bars)
- Smoking cessation assistance
- Evaluating components of bans
- Reduction in active smoking and increased smoking cessation secondary to the ban

Secondhand Smoke Exposure

Before Ban:
- Variable exposures depending upon individual sources of secondhand smoke exposure (e.g., living with a smoker, work in smoking environments, time in vehicles with smoke) or existing smoking regulations in certain venues
- Potential for chronic exposures or intermittent exposures (e.g., weekly exposures when an individual goes out once a week to a smoky bar)

After Ban:
- Exposure varies depending upon individual sources of secondhand-smoke exposure (e.g., possibility of controlled smoke exposure at home, in cars, bars, and other areas where smoking is allowed after the ban)
- Impact of individual exposures on secondhand smokers
- Impact of individual exposures on smokers

Potential Health Outcomes

Before Ban:
- Acute coronary events triggered by short-term secondhand-smoke exposure
- Subclinical conditions mediated by chronic exposure to secondhand smoke that predispose an individual to acute coronary events

After Ban:
- Decreases in the number of acute coronary events triggered by short-term or longer-term (e.g., full work day at office) secondhand-smoke exposure
- Gradual decrease in the number of individuals with subclinical conditions or in the severity of the subclinical conditions that predispose an individual to an acute coronary event due to decreased chronic exposure to secondhand smoke
- Decreases in both the number of acute coronary events and predisposing conditions in smokers from decreased number of smokers and decreased number of cigarettes smoked by smokers

FIGURE 1-1 Factors that can affect the impact of smoking bans on cardiovascular outcomes. A number of policy-related variables can differ among locations and affect the impact of a smoking ban. The concentration of secondhand smoke can also differ among locations both before and after a ban is implemented. Outcome-related factors can differ and affect study results.

cessation.[2] Second, not all the key publications quantified the extent to which the smoking bans resulted in a decrease in secondhand-smoke exposure. Third, partial smoking bans were in place in some areas before the bans examined in the studies and would have decreased secondhand-smoke exposure prior to the implementation of the law. Exposure issues related to secondhand smoke are discussed in detail in Chapter 2, and the specific exposure measurements used in the key studies are discussed in Chapter 6. Another concern is the assessment of exposure to secondhand smoke itself. There is a hierarchy of exposure-assessment methods, and most of the studies use different methods; although some of the studies are strong in assessment (for example, using measurements of secondhand smoke before and after the implementation of a ban), others are not as rigorous. Exposure assessment in general is discussed in Chapter 2 and assessment in the individual studies in Chapter 6. The issue of exposure is further complicated by the potential effects of acute versus chronic exposures. As seen in Figure 1-1, in the key studies examining smoking bans secondhand-smoke exposure could be chronic or intermittent prior to a smoking ban being implemented. After a smoking ban, chronic or intermittent exposures could still occur but possibly to a lesser extent because of the ban (see Chapter 2 for a discussion of the effect of a ban on secondhand smoke exposures). Similarly, in cohort and case–control studies the exposures could be chronic or intermittent. Because the duration, frequency and magnitude of the exposures are not analyzed in many of those studies, most of the conclusions of the committee are made for exposure in general, assuming some recurrent level of recurrent secondhand-smoke exposure. Acute, chronic, and intermittent exposures have been evaluated in experimental studies, which can provide information on the duration of exposure required to produce an effect. Those studies address the pathophysiology of any cardiovascular effects and the timeframes associated with any effects.

The issue of the interval between implementation of a smoking ban and a change in the rate of acute coronary events is included in the charge to the committee (Question 5) and is relevant to the committee's judgment as to the biologic plausibility of a relationship between exposure to secondhand smoke and acute coronary events. That period is difficult to define under circumstances in which the precise date of initiation of an intervention is not known and can vary within an area, depending on compliance and enforcement. The time period is relevant to the mechanisms by which secondhand smoke could cause acute coronary events. The committee also examined time between exposure to particulate matter and cardiovascular

---

[2] The distinction between effects in nonsmokers and effects in smokers is important for assessing the effects of secondhand-smoke exposure on acute coronary events, but not for assessing the effects of smoking bans on acute coronary events.

effects because particulate matter is a component of secondhand smoke. This issue is discussed in Chapter 2 and, with regard to the key studies, in Chapter 7.

The key studies used two types of controls. With one type, a study compared acute cardiovascular events in a given population before and during a smoking ban. (One study also investigated what happened when a ban was lifted.) Such a study cannot evaluate the effects of other changes over time (when, in all the areas involved, both rates of smoking and rates of acute cardiovascular disease were generally going down). Other studies instead (or in addition) selected as a control population people in an area that did not implement a ban. A study of that design can to some extent control for larger trends (secular trends), but inevitably such comparison populations could differ from study populations in several ways that might be related to both the likelihood of exposure to secondhand smoke and the incidence of acute cardiovascular events, and this would add uncertainty to the results of the study. Issues related to controls are discussed in Chapter 7.

An important aspect of the committee's charge to weigh the evidence of a causal association between secondhand-smoke exposure and acute coronary events is the biologic plausibility of the association. Evidence related to biologic plausibility comes from experimental studies of humans and other animals. Because air pollution has many of the same constituents as secondhand smoke, the committee also reviewed evidence of a relationship between air pollution and acute coronary events. That information is discussed in Chapter 3.

The key studies discussed in this report are necessarily nonexperimental; they are observational or surveillance studies that looked at the effect of a smoking ban on hospital outcomes, out-of-hospital deaths, or both. Nonexperimental design can result in decreased information on the individual level, including information on exposure and in some instances smoking status. The results of population-based smoking-ban studies can be part of the evidence of a causal relationship between secondhand smoke and acute coronary events.

Other considerations in the determination of causality historically have included temporality, strength of the association, dose–response relationship, identified biologic mechanism, specificity, coherence with existing theory and knowledge, experimental evidence, and alternate explanations. Population-based studies can provide some evidence related to most of those, but they cannot yield experimental evidence and cannot rule out all alternative explanations. The epidemiologic studies under consideration are not randomized controlled studies, so they are subject to several potential sources of bias and confounding that need to be taken into account in weighing the validity of their results. Each of the studies has strengths, limitations, and weaknesses, including standard epidemiologic limitations related to time-trend studies, comparison groups, control of confounding factors, lack of individual biologic measurements, and information on concurrent efforts.

Another important aspect to consider is the hypothesis tested in a study. A study could try to test several hypotheses related to secondhand-smoke exposure; each hypothesis might be best answered with a different study design, and each would be related to different questions being asked of this committee. A cohort study could test the hypothesis that long-term exposure to secondhand smoke increases the risk of coronary events, a "natural experimental" study could test the hypothesis that a long-term reduction in secondhand-smoke exposure leads to a reduced incidence of events, and an observational case-crossover study with detailed examination of the temporal relationships between exposure and episodes and detailed exposure assessment (a study similar, for example, to time-series studies of air pollution that looked at the relationship between exposures and acute coronary events) could be used to test the hypothesis that secondhand-smoke exposure triggers acute coronary events in people who are at risk. Each type of study answers different questions that are integrated into the charge to this committee.

Additional problems in using population-based studies like these when trying to infer causality include the inability to assess the pathophysiology of a relationship between secondhand-smoke exposure and acute cardiac events, difficulty in assessing dose–response relationships, and difficulty in determining the strength of a relationship in the absence of subgroup analyses of smokers, nonsmokers, and people with greater or smaller magnitudes of other risk factors. Experimental data provide information on the pathophysiology and on dose–response relationships.

Most of the studies assume a linear trend variable (month) to quantify secular trends in the rate of acute coronary events, and some of these (Juster et al., 2007; Khuder et al., 2007) fit a linear-regression model that yields an estimated age- and sex-adjusted rate of an adverse outcome. The committee discusses those approaches and other aspects related to the statistical analysis in Chapter 7.

ORGANIZATION OF THIS REPORT

This remainder of this report is organized into seven chapters and one appendix. Chapter 2 summarizes the data on exposure to secondhand smoke, including its constituents, its measurement, and typical exposure to it in the absence and presence of smoking bans. Chapter 3 presents studies of pathophysiologic responses to secondhand-smoke exposure that could be related to cardiovascular effects. It summarizes information from cellular, animal, and human experimental studies, and presents conclusions and recommendations based on the surgeon general's 2006 report and other research. Epidemiologic studies that looked at the association between secondhand-smoke exposure and cardiovascular disease and acute coronary events, other than studies related to smoking bans, are discussed in Chapter 4. Chapter 5 contains background on the history and context of smoking bans around the world. Chapter 6 describes the 11 key studies that examined acute coronary events in relation to smoking bans, focusing on data sources, study design, the choice of end points, and possible confounders. The information from those key studies as well as the pathophysiologic data and other epidemiologic studies discussed in Chapter 4 are then synthesized in Chapter 7. In Chapter 8, the committee summarizes its conclusions about the association between secondhand-smoke exposure and cardiovascular disease, secondhand-smoke exposure and acute coronary events, and smoking bans and acute coronary events, discussing the weight of evidence for the associations. In that chapter the committee also presents its responses to the specific questions outlined in Box 1-1. The appendix presents agendas of the public meetings held by the committee.

REFERENCES

AHA (American Heart Association). 2009. (Accessed April 6, 2009, from http://www.americanheart.org/presenter.jhtml?identifier=4741).

Barone-Adesi, F., L. Vizzini, F. Merletti, and L. Richiardi. 2006. Short-term effects of Italian smoking regulation on rates of hospital admission for acute myocardial infarction. *European Heart Journal* 27(20):2468-2472.

Bartecchi, C., R. N. Alsever, C. Nevin-Woods, W. M. Thomas, R. O. Estacio, B. B. Bartelson, and M. J. Krantz. 2006. Reduction in the incidence of acute myocardial infarction associated with a citywide smoking ordinance. *Circulation* 114(14):1490-1496.

Cal EPA (California Environmental Protection Agency). 2005a. *Proposed identification of environmental tobacco smoke as a toxic air contaminant. Part A: Exposure assessment.* Sacramento, CA: California Environmental Protection Agency.

———. 2005b. *Proposed identification of environmental tobacco smoke as a toxic air contaminant. Part B: Health effects.* Sacramento, CA: California Environmental Protection Agency.

CDC (Centers for Disease Control and Prevention). 2009. Reduced hospitalizations for acute myocardial infarction after implementation of a smoke-free ordinance—city of Pueblo, Colorado, 2002–2006. *MMWR—Morbidity & Mortality Weekly Report* 57(51):1373-1377.

Cesaroni, G., F. Forastiere, N. Agabiti, P. Valente, P. Zuccaro, and C. A. Perucci. 2008. Effect of the Italian smoking ban on population rates of acute coronary events. *Circulation* 117(9):1183-1188.

Critchley, J. A., and S. Capewell. 2003. Mortality risk reduction associated with smoking cessation in patients with coronary heart disease: A systematic review. *JAMA* 290(1):86-97.

Dobson, A. J., H. M. Alexander, R. F. Heller, and D. M. Lloyd. 1991. How soon after quitting smoking does risk of heart attack decline? *Journal of Clinical Epidemiology* 44(11):1247-1253.

Doll, R., and R. Peto. 1976. Mortality in relation to smoking: 20 years' observations on male British doctors. *British Medical Journal* 2(6051):1525-1536.

Gordon, T., W. B. Kannel, D. McGee, and T. R. Dawber. 1974. Death and coronary attacks in men after giving up cigarette smoking. A report from the Framingham Study. *Lancet* 2(7893):1345-1348.

HHS (U.S. Department of Health and Human Services). 1972. *The health consequences of smoking.* Rockville, MD: U.S. Department of Health and Human Services, Centers for Disease Control and Prevention, National Center for Chronic Disease Prevention and Health Promotion, Office on Smoking and Health.

———. 1986. *The health consequences of involuntary smoking: A report of the surgeon general.* Rockville, MD: U.S. Department of Health and Human Services, Centers for Disease Control and Prevention, National Center for Chronic Disease Prevention and Health Promotion, Office on Smoking and Health.

———. 1990. *The health benefits of smoking cessation: A report of the surgeon general.* Atlanta, GA: U.S. Department of Health and Human Services, Centers for Disease Control and Prevention, Coordinating Center for Health Promotion, National Center for Chronic Disease Prevention and Health Promotion, Office on Smoking and Health.

———. 2000. *Healthy people 2010. 2nd ed. With understanding and improving health and objectives for improving health. 2 vols.* Washington, DC: U.S. Government Printing Office.

———. 2005. *Report on carcinogens. 11th ed.* U.S. Department of Health and Human Services, Public Health Service, National Toxicology Program.

———. 2006. *The health consequences of involuntary exposure to tobacco smoke: A report of the surgeon general.* Atlanta, GA: U.S. Department of Health and Human Services, Centers for Disease Control and Prevention, Coordinating Center for Health Promotion, National Center for Chronic Disease Prevention and Health Promotion, Office on Smoking and Health.

IOM (Institute of Medicine). 2007. *Ending the tobacco problem: A blueprint for the nation.* Washington, DC: The National Academies Press.

Juster, H. R., B. R. Loomis, T. M. Hinman, M. C. Farrelly, A. Hyland, U. E. Bauer, and G. S. Birkhead. 2007. Declines in hospital admissions for acute myocardial infarction in New York state after implementation of a comprehensive smoking ban. *American Journal of Public Health* 97(11):2035-2039.

Khuder, S. A., S. Milz, T. Jordan, J. Price, K. Silvestri, and P. Butler. 2007. The impact of a smoking ban on hospital admissions for coronary heart disease. *Preventive Medicine* 45(1):3-8.

Lemstra, M., C. Neudorf, and J. Opondo. 2008. Implications of a public smoking ban. *Canadian Journal of Public Health* 99(1):62-65.

Lightwood, J. M., and S. A. Glantz. 1997. Short-term economic and health benefits of smoking cessation: Myocardial infarction and stroke. *Circulation* 96(4):1089-1096.

Lightwood, J. M., P. G. Coxson, K. Bibbins-Domingo, L. W. Williams, and L. Goldman. 2009. Coronary heart disease attributable to passive smoking: CHD policy model. *American Journal of Preventive Medicine* 36(1):13-20.

NCI (National Cancer Institute). 1997. *Monograph 8: Changes in cigarette-related disease risks and their implications for prevention and control.* Bethesda, MD: National Institutes of Health.

Negri, E., C. La Vecchia, B. D'Avanzo, A. Nobili, and R. G. La Malfa. 1994. Acute myocardial infarction: Association with time since stopping smoking in Italy. GISSI-EFRIM investigators. Gruppo Italiano per lo Studio della Sopravvivenza nell'infarto. Epidemiologia dei Fattori di Rischio dell'Infarto Miocardico. *Journal of Epidemiology and Community Health* 48(2):129-133.

Pell, J. P., S. Haw, S. Cobbe, D. E. Newby, A. C. H. Pell, C. Fischbacher, A. McConnachie, S. Pringle, D. Murdoch, F. Dunn, K. Oldroyd, P. Macintyre, B. O'Rourke, and W. Borland. 2008. Smoke-free legislation and hospitalizations for acute coronary syndrome. *New England Journal of Medicine* 359(5):482-491.

Pirkle, J. L., K. M. Flegal, J. T. Bernert, D. J. Brody, R. A. Etzel, and K. R. Maurer. 1996. Exposure of the US population to environmental tobacco smoke: The third National Health and Nutrition Examination Survey, 1988 to 1991. *JAMA* 275(16):1233-1240.

Sargent, R. P., R. M. Shepard, and S. A. Glantz. 2004. Reduced incidence of admissions for myocardial infarction associated with public smoking ban: Before and after study. *BMJ* 328(7446):977-980.

Seo, D.-C., and M. R. Torabi. 2007. Reduced admissions for acute myocardial infarction associated with a public smoking ban: Matched controlled study. *Journal of Drug Education* 37(3):217-226.

Teo, K. K., S. Ounpuu, S. Hawken, M. R. Pandey, V. Valentin, D. Hunt, R. Diaz, W. Rashed, R. Freeman, L. Jiang, X. Zhang, S. Yusuf, and I. S. Investigators. 2006. Tobacco use and risk of myocardial infarction in 52 countries in the INTERHEART study: A case-control study. *Lancet* 368(9536):647-658.

Vasselli, S., P. Papini, D. Gaelone, L. Spizzichino, E. De Campora, R. Gnavi, C. Saitto, N. Binkin, and G. Laurendi. 2008. Reduction incidence of myocardial infarction associated with a national legislative ban on smoking. *Minerva Cardioangiologica* 56(2):197-203.

2

Evaluating Exposure to Secondhand Smoke

Important considerations in evaluating the effects of secondhand smoke include the magnitude of exposure to it,[1] how exposure can be measured, and how exposure changes with the implementation of smoking bans. This chapter discusses the constituents of secondhand smoke and the measurement of exposure to secondhand smoke, beginning with measurement of airborne tracers of secondhand smoke and of its main biologic markers (or biomarkers)—the nicotine metabolite cotinine and metabolites of 4-(methylnitrosamino)-1-(3-pyridyl)-1-butanone (NNK). It then summarizes the information available on secondhand-smoke concentrations and exposures before and after the implementation of smoking bans.

CONSTITUENTS OF SECONDHAND SMOKE

Cigarette smoke is a complex aerosol[2] consisting of thousands of chemicals (Cal EPA, 2005b). It consists of gases and volatile chemicals in which particulate matter (PM) is suspended. The gas phase consists of air, carbon dioxide, carbon monoxide, and many other chemicals, including nicotine, carbonyls (such as acetaldehyde, formaldehyde, and acrolein), hydrocarbons (such as benzene, toluene, and some polycyclic aromatic hydrocarbons

---

[1] For the purpose of this report, the committee defined secondhand smoke as a complex mixture that is made up of gases and particles and includes smoke from burning cigarettes, cigars, and pipe tobacco (sidestream smoke) and exhaled mainstream smoke (CDC, 2006). This includes aged smoke that lingers after smoking ceases.

[2] An aerosol is a suspension of solid or liquid particles in a gas, and includes both the particles and the suspending gas (Hinds, 1999).

[PAHs]), nitrogen oxides, pyridine, ammonia, nitrosamines, and hydrogen cyanide (Cal EPA, 2005b). The particulate phase, "tar," consists of thousands more chemicals, including alkaloids, larger PAHs, tobacco-specific nitrosamines, polonium-210, nickel, cadmium, arsenic, and lead. Some compounds, such as cresols and PAHs, are partitioned between vapor and particulate phases.

About 85% of secondhand smoke is composed of sidestream smoke emerging from the burning tip of the cigarette and the remainder is exhaled in mainstream smoke (the smoke inhaled by a smoker when puffing on a cigarette) (Kritz et al., 1995). The measured sidestream emissions of chemicals are quite similar among a wide range of cigarette brands and styles, including regular, unfiltered, filtered, and "low tar, low nicotine" cigarettes.[3] Although the composition of sidestream and mainstream smoke are qualitatively similar, there are substantial quantitative differences in composition between mainstream and sidestream smoke because the chemicals emitted in tobacco smoke change with temperature, oxygen concentration, pH, and the extent of combustion.[4] Those factors are different in mainstream and sidestream smoke (Jenkins et al., 2000). As summarized elsewhere, most compounds from cigarettes are emitted in sidestream smoke in much higher amounts than in mainstream smoke (Cal EPA, 2005a; Jenkins et al., 2000; NRC, 1986). For instance, the ratio of the mass of benzene emitted into sidestream smoke compared to that emitted into mainstream smoke is approximately 10, while the corresponding ratio for the 4-aminobiphenyl is 30, and that, for nicotine is approximately 2. More recently, Lodovici et al. (2004) reported that the amount of total PAH in sidestream smoke "was about tenfold higher compared with mainstream smoke." Nicotine is primarily in the particulate phase of mainstream smoke but predominantly in the vapor phase in secondhand smoke (Cal EPA, 2005a). This variable ratio from compound to compound between sidestream and mainstream smoke makes it impossible to characterize a passive smoking exposure as a simple fraction of the dose a smoker receives; such a comparison must be chemical specific (Hammond et al., 1993). Thus, while on average nonsmokers exposed to secondhand smoke have about 1% the cotinine (a metabolite of nicotine) as smokers, they have 14% as much 4-aminobiphenyl (a potent human carcinogen) adducted to their hemoglobin (Hammond et al., 1993).

---

[3] The variability in mainstream smoke among these designs is due to the ventilation holes in some cigarettes; the ventilation dilutes the mainstream smoke when tested on cigarette machines, but not when smoked by smokers. The resultant variability in reported mainstream emissions among these cigarettes results in wide ranges in reported ratios of sidestream to mainstream smoke emissions, despite the consistency in the sidestream emissions.

[4] Inhaling through the cigarette draws air to the burning end of the cigarette so that it burns hotter (just as embers in a wood stove burn hotter and turn red when air is blown on them) as it has more oxygen than when the burning tip is smoldering.

Animal experiments by Philip Morris laboratories have demonstrated that sidestream smoke is three to four times more toxic than mainstream smoke (Schick and Glantz, 2005).

This complex picture becomes even more complicated over time. The ambient emissions from cigarettes can undergo further chemical reactions and deposit at varying rates on surfaces (Jenkins et al., 2000). For example, chemical analyses of aging sidestream smoke have shown that the carcinogenic nitrosamine NNK can form from nicotine and increase over time (Schick and Glantz, 2007). The chemical and physical properties of PM in secondhand tobacco smoke also change rapidly due, for example, to diffusion and coagulation, particle setting and impaction, and chemical reactions (Benner et al., 1989; Eatough et al., 1989); however, measurements of concentrations in smoking environments averaged over a day to a week have demonstrated similar ratios of PM to nicotine (Daisey, 1999; Leaderer and Hammond, 1991).

The toxicity of sidestream smoke appears to increase over time. Schick and Glantz (2006), using data from a series of inhalation experiments in rats conducted at Philip Morris, compared freshly generated sidestream smoke to sidestream smoke that had been aged for 30–90 minutes in a 30 m^3 chamber. When the smoke doses were equalized on the basis of particulate material concentration, aged sidestream smoke was four times more toxic in 21-day exposures and two times more toxic in 90-day exposures than the freshly generated sidestream smoke. Moreover, current methodologic limitations prevent estimation of concentrations of highly reactive compounds; this is particularly important for the more reactive constituents of tobacco smoke and for estimating their concentrations in secondhand smoke dispersed in an unspecified space. A partial list of cigarette smoke constituents in mainstream and sidestream smoke in amounts exceeding 10 μg/per cigarette is presented in Table 2-1.

MEASUREMENT OF SECONDHAND SMOKE

Tobacco smoke is a complex mixture of thousands of compounds. The composition of secondhand smoke changes over time; substances emitted from cigarettes can undergo chemical reactions and deposit on surfaces at various rates (Singer et al., 2002). Several approaches to evaluating and comparing human exposures to secondhand smoke, including measurement of airborne tracers or biomarkers of exposure (see Table 2-2), are useful.

In a 1986 report (NRC, 1986) on secondhand smoke (or environmental tobacco smoke, ETS), the National Research Council stated that "a marker or tracer for quantifying ETS concentrations should be:

- unique or nearly unique to the tobacco smoke so that other sources are minor in comparison,
- a constituent of the tobacco smoke present in sufficient quantity such that concentrations of it can be easily detected in air, even at low smoking rates,
- similar in emission rates for a variety of tobacco products, and
- in a fairly consistent ratio to the individual contaminant of interest or category of contaminants of interest (e.g., suspended particulates) under a range of environmental conditions encountered and for a variety of tobacco products."

Those criteria remain important today. In a recent report (2006), the National Research Council presented similar criteria that should be considered in selecting a biomarker, regardless of its intended use. The criteria include the sensitivity of the assay for the biomarker, the specificity of the

TABLE 2-1 Amount of Cigarette Smoke Constituents in Tobacco Smoke and Smoking Environments. Partial List of the Cigarette Smoke Constituents Generated in Mainstream and Secondhand Smoke in Amounts Exceeding 10 μg per Cigarette or That Have Been Shown to Be Cardiotoxic

Compound	Average Amount (μg per cigarette except where noted)	Present in Secondhand Smoke (>10 μg per cigarette)	Mean Concentration in Smoking Environments
Carbon dioxide	30,000		
Carbon monoxide	20,000	Yes	0.2–33 ppm[a]
Nicotine	1,650	Yes	0.6–106 μg/m^{3a}
Acetaldehyde	700		370–462 μg/m^{3a}
Acetic acid	570		
Hydrogen cyanide	450		
Formic acid	340		
Nitrogen oxides	300		3–350 ppb[a]
Formaldehyde	300	Yes	5–1,100 μg/m^{3a}
Methyl chloride	300		
Benzene[b]	30	Yes	2–100 μg/m^{3a}
Acetone	250		
Catechol	195		
1,3-butadiene[c]	150	Yes	0.2–19 μg/m^{3a}
Toluene	150		
Methanol	135		
Hydroquinone	120		
Lactic acid	120		

TABLE 2-1 Continued

Compound	Average Amount (μg per cigarette except where noted)	Present in Secondhand Smoke (>10 μg per cigarette)	Mean Concentration in Smoking Environments
Succinic acid	120		
Phenol	100		
Ammonia	100		
Glycolic acid	100		
4-vinylcatechol	84		
Acrolein[c]	80	Yes	14–100 $\mu g/m^{3a}$
Methylethylketone	70		
3-cresol	60		
4-cresol	60		
Propionaldehyde	45		25–110 $\mu g/m^{3a}$
Resorcinol	44		
3-methylfluoranthene	40		
4-methylcatechol	38		
3-methylcatechol	38		
4-vinylphenol	30		
2-methylfluranthene	30		
Pyridine	30		1.34–6.5 $\mu g/m^{3a}$
Carbon disulfide	30	Yes	
4-ethylcatechol	28		
3-picoline	24		
4-picoline	24		
2-cresol	22		
3-vinylpyridine	22	Yes	
Cholesterol	22		
Benzoic acid	20		
3-ethylphenol	18		
4-ethylphenol	18		
Crotonaldehyde	15	Yes	
2-methoxyphenol	13		
2-picoline	12		
Butyraldehyde	12	Yes	
4-vinylguaiacol	11		
Cadmium[c]	0.5	Yes	3–10 $ng/m^{3d,e}$
Lead[c]	0.4	Yes	
Benzo[a]pyrene	0.075	Yes	0.4–22 ng/m^{3a}
Chromium[c]	0.07		1.2–8.9 ng/m^{3a}
Nickel[c]	0.05		2.5–7.2 ng/m^{3a}
Particulate matter	50[f]	Yes	27–2,000 $\mu g/m^{3a}$

[a] Data are from Jenkins et al., 1999.

[b] Benzene concentration present in sidestream smoke is 163–353 μg per cigarette.

[c] Amount is for sidestream smoke.

[d] Data are from Bolte et al., 2008.

[e] Data are from Brauer and Mannetje, 1998.

[f] The concentration of particulate matter is in $\mu m/m^3$.

TABLE 2-2 Biomarkers and Airborne Tracers

	Advantages	Disadvantages
Biomarkers	Dose; integrates exposures from all sources	Does not distinguish source location
Nicotine in body fluids	Specific to tobacco	Very short half-life in fluids (therefore only measures exposure that occurred in previous few hours)
Nicotine in hair, nails	Specific to tobacco Easy, noninvasive to collect Reflects longer period of exposure	Does not indicate recent exposures or patterns of exposure
Cotinine in body fluids	Specific to tobacco Easy, noninvasive to collect in saliva, urine Sensitive (present in high levels so easy to detect low-level exposure)	Short half-life in fluids, so measures recent exposure (only the previous few days) Blood samples are more invasive to collect
NNK metabolites	Specific to tobacco Can detect in urine Longer half-life in fluids relative to nicotine (therefore can measure exposure over several weeks)	Expensive (greater analytical costs for assay)
Airborne Tracers	Measures and compares exposures from different sources (for example, in different venues such as homes, workplaces, and public places)	Requires measurement of all sources to determine exposures from all sources Does not reflect individual respiratory rates

biomarker for the chemical or metabolite of interest, the relevance of the biomarker to the exposure and disease outcome of interest, the practicality of the biomarker (both in the ability to collect a biologic sample and in the analytic method), and the pharmacokinetics of the biomarkers, especially in terms of its half-life of the compound measured. Although few, if any, biomarkers have been shown to meet all the criteria, a number of biomarkers of secondhand-smoke exposure that meet many of the criteria are available.

Measures of exposure in the air and of biomarkers of exposure are complementary. Assuming equally accurate and sensitive methods, bio-

TABLE 2-2 Continued

	Advantages	Disadvantages
Airborne NNK	Specific to tobacco smoke Of intrinsic health interest (known carcinogen)	Expensive (greater analytical costs for assay) Less sensitive than nicotine because present in lower concentration (therefore can not measure as low secondhand smoke concentrations)
Particulate matter	Present at high levels in secondhand smoke so can measure a wide range of concentrations relatively easily Can measure with continuous sampler and get information directly, without laboratory	Not specific to tobacco smoke and many other sources present at all times, therefore not distinguishable from other sources of PM at lower secondhand-smoke concentrations Initial investment in equipment expensive, but little operating cost
Airborne Nicotine	Specific to tobacco smoke Of intrinsic health interest (known cardiovascular agent) Present at high levels in secondhand smoke facilitating easy measurement of a wide range of concentrations, including very low concentrations	Different decay rate than other secondhand smoke constituents, so complicates estimation of exposure to those other constituents Requires laboratory analyses

Abbreviations: NNK, 4-(methylnitrosamino)-1-(3-pyridyl)-1-butanone.

markers afford better measurement of the dose that a person receives because they integrate all sources of exposure and reflect inhalation rates, which might vary from person to person and for a given person over time. Interpretation of the level of a biomarker, however, must consider its half-life: if its half-life is short, only recent exposure is measured. Airborne tracers of exposure are able to show the relative contributions of different sources or venues of an exposure (for example, home exposures compared with workplace exposures). In contrast, biomarkers do not differentiate between sources of exposure but rather integrate all exposures and reflect true dose.

Airborne Tracers of Secondhand Smoke

Nicotine and its metabolite cotinine have been widely used as tracers of secondhand smoke. Ambient nicotine can be measured accurately and sensitively, and cotinine can be measured in saliva, blood, and urine. One major characteristic that contributes to the widespread use of airborne nicotine and cotinine is that tobacco is virtually the only source of both compounds, so they meet the criterion noted earlier. Furthermore, tobacco smoke contains large amounts of nicotine, so tobacco smoke can be detected even at low concentrations. Sensitive, specific, and accurate methods to measure nicotine in ambient air and cotinine in body fluids are now well established and have been used in dozens of investigations around the world.

Another commonly used tracer for secondhand smoke is particulate matter (PM). In heavy-smoking environments—such as bars, pubs, and many restaurants—the concentration of PM can be extremely high, and direct-reading instruments provide immediate data without the need for a laboratory. However, there are many other sources of PM, which is ubiquitous, so that even if no smoking occurs, PM is present at levels that might affect health, as is known from air-pollution studies. This background level of PM complicates measurement of PM from secondhand smoke at low secondhand-smoke levels. Because virtually all secondhand-smoke particles are less than 2.5 micrometers in diameter, all secondhand-smoke particles are contained in $PM_{2.5}$, and eliminating particles larger than 2.5 micrometers, for example, by the use of an impactor or other size selector, reduces the contribution of non-secondhand-smoke PM (Cal EPA, 2005a). That does not, however, eliminate the PM from traffic or other combustion sources.

Nicotine and some other components of secondhand smoke deposit readily onto surfaces, with very small amounts of re-emission. Highly volatile gases in secondhand smoke (such as benzene and butadiene) tend not to deposit on surfaces. A few hours after smoking has ceased, most of the airborne nicotine will have deposited on surfaces, but nearly all the benzene and butadiene will remain in the air (Singer et al., 2002). If nicotine is used as the only tracer for those other gases, and the ratio of nicotine to benzene in fresh smoke is used to estimate the benzene concentration, one may underestimate the exposure of room occupants to benzene. That is true for many other toxic chemicals in secondhand smoke, and this drawback applies to the use of cotinine as a biomarker as well as to nicotine as a tracer in the air. Despite the limitation, airborne nicotine and cotinine remain extremely useful in evaluating exposures in many settings.

Biomarkers of Exposure to Secondhand Smoke

Although most of the toxicants in tobacco smoke are not specific to tobacco-smoke exposure, because they are generic products of combustion of organic materials, two toxicants—nicotine and NNK—are peculiar to tobacco smoke and are known to have adverse health effects. Those compounds or their metabolites can be measured with high sensitivity in various biologic matrices in people exposed to secondhand smoke. Although a number of other tobacco-smoke constituents—such as carbon monoxide, acrolein, benzene, and PAHs and their metabolites—have been used as biomarkers of exposure for active smokers, they are not good biomarkers of exposure to secondhand smoke because they are not unique to secondhand smoke and are present at low levels compared to other sources. Their concentrations in active smokers exceed concentrations seen in most nonsmokers, but secondhand smoke contributes only small amounts of them relative to background amounts (for example, from exposures in food and air pollution).

Nicotine and Its Metabolites

Nicotine is present in substantial concentrations in all tobacco products. It is also present in some foods, but the concentrations are much lower, and the contribution of food to the body burden of nicotine and its metabolites is insignificant (Benowitz, 1999). Once nicotine is in the body, hepatic enzymes metabolize it extensively (see Figure 2-1). Nicotine is converted to cotinine, which is converted to *trans*-3'-hydroxycotinine (3-HC) by the hepatic enzyme cytochrome P450 2A6 (CYP450 2A6) (Hukkanen et al., 2005). Nicotine, cotinine, and 3-HC are converted to their glucuronide metabolites by various uridine diphosphate-glucuronosyl transferase (UGT) enzymes. Cotinine is the major proximate metabolite of nicotine. On average, about 70–80% of nicotine is converted to cotinine, primarily by the liver enzyme CYP450 2A6 (Hukkanen et al., 2005).

Cotinine can be measured in blood, saliva, urine, hair, toenails, and other biologic fluids. The average half-life of cotinine (16 h) in plasma is longer than that of nicotine (2 h). Therefore, cotinine concentrations are more stable throughout the day, and this makes it the preferred biomarker of smoke exposure in blood, saliva, and urine. Both nicotine and cotinine are persistent in hair and toenails. Concentrations of cotinine in blood (including plasma and serum) and saliva are highly correlated and similar. Urinary cotinine concentrations, however, are on average 4–5 times higher than those in blood or saliva, so urine is a more sensitive matrix for detection of low exposure (Benowitz et al., 2009).

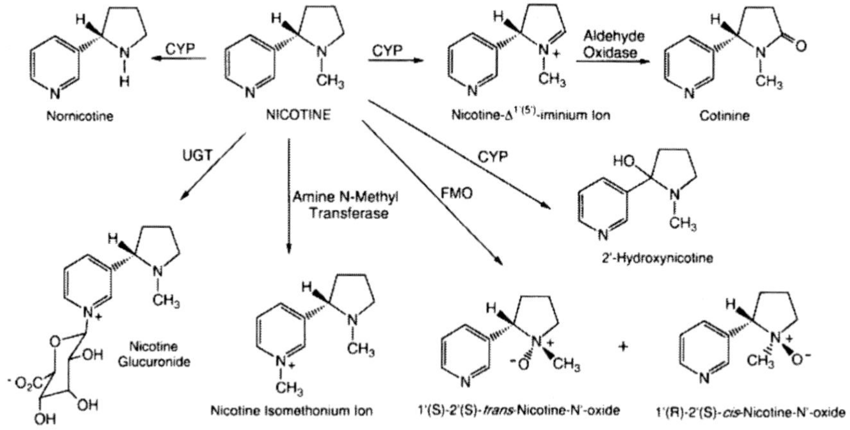

FIGURE 2-1 Primary routes of nicotine metabolism. The figure shows the major routes of nicotine metabolism, with the majority of nicotine being metabolized to cotinine via CYP and aldehyde oxidase. Abbreviations: CYP, cytochrome P450; FMO, flavin-containing monooxygenase; UGT, uridine diphosphate-glucuronosyltransferase. SOURCE: Hukkanen et al., 2005.

Nicotine is excreted in urine as various metabolites (see Figure 2-1). Excreted nicotine, cotinine, and 3-HC and their glucuronide conjugates account for about 85–90% of a nicotine dose (Hukkanen et al., 2005). Measuring the sum of the metabolites provides a reasonably precise estimate of daily nicotine dose and is the gold standard for biomarker assessment of nicotine exposure.

Interindividual variability in the rate and pattern of nicotine and cotinine metabolism affects the concentration of cotinine that results from a given exposure to nicotine. Factors that may influence nicotine metabolism include genetic variation, race, sex, use of oral contraceptives or other estrogen-containing hormones, renal failure, and use of various medications, such as anticonvulsants and rifampin (Hukkanen et al., 2005). Despite that, cotinine levels are useful to differentiate smokers from nonsmokers, to categorize nonsmokers into groups with varying levels of exposure to secondhand smoke, and to track changes in population exposure to secondhand smoke.

NNK Metabolites

NNK is a nicotine-derived nitrosamine that is a potent carcinogen. It is formed primarily in the tobacco-curing process, during which nicotine or pseudo-oxynicotine reacts with nitrite in tobacco (Hecht, 2004). NNK is metabolized in the body to 4-(N-nitrosomethylamino)-1-(3-pyridyl)-1-butanol (NNAL) and NNAL-glucuronides, which are excreted in urine. NNAL and NNAL-glucuronides are commonly measured together and termed total NNAL. NNAL remains in the body much longer than cotinine, with a terminal half-life of about 3 weeks, so it might be usable for assessing secondhand-smoke exposure over a longer period than cotinine. Although urinary NNAL is sensitive and specific as a biomarker of secondhand-smoke exposure, no studies have evaluated the relationship between urinary NNAL concentration and cardiovascular disease.

EXPOSURES TO SECONDHAND SMOKE

General Trends in Exposure to Secondhand Smoke

Nicotine concentrations measured in diverse environments that allow smoking range over 4 orders of magnitude, from less than 0.1 $\mu g/m^3$ to several hundred $\mu g/m^3$. The weekly average concentrations measured in the homes of smokers is typically 0.5–5 $\mu g/m^3$, with a median of 1 $\mu g/m^3$ and a mean of 2.2 $\mu g/m^3$ (Leaderer and Hammond, 1991). The 1 week average nicotine concentrations found in 279 low-income homes with smokers was 3.3 $\mu g/m^3$ (Emmons et al., 2001). A similar average weekly value, 3.7 $\mu g/m^3$, was found in the homes of 103 low-income children in Colorado where there were smokers but no strict smoking bans (Wamboldt et al., 2008). One-week sampling of 49 low-income, multi-family homes (including smoking and nonsmoking homes) in the Greater Boston Area found nicotine concentrations ranging from below the limit of detection to 26.92 $\mu g/m^3$ (Kraev et al., 2009). Clearly secondhand-smoke exposure in the homes of smokers remains high in some cases. The mean and median concentrations were 2.2 and 0.13 $\mu g/m^3$, respectively, and the concentration was associated with the number of smokers residing in the unit and the number of cigarettes smoked in the home as reported on a questionnaire. Workplace and restaurant concentrations can be over 10 $\mu g/m^3$, bars over 20 $\mu g/m^3$, and discotheques over 100 $\mu g/m^3$ (Hammond, 1999). In a recent study of nine homes with smoking and three smoke-free homes in the United States, $PM_{2.5}$ measured in real time over a 3-day period averaged 84 $\mu g/m^3$ in the primary smoking area of the smoking houses, 63 $\mu g/m^3$ in a distal area from the primary smoking area, and 9 $\mu g/m^3$ in the nonsmoking homes (Van Deusen et al., 2009).

Over the past 25 years, smoking restrictions and bans in the United States in workplaces, restaurants, and other public places have been increasing, both voluntarily and because of regulations. Their efficacy is seen at the national level in the United States in the 70% decrease in serum cotinine concentrations in 14 years. The data in Figure 2-2 are from the

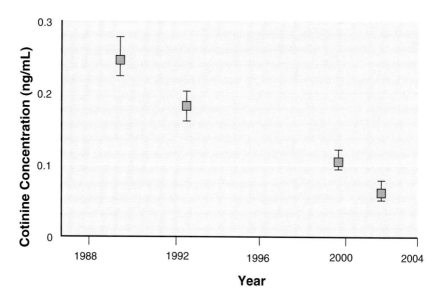

FIGURE 2-2 Serum cotinine in nonsmokers in the United States exposed to secondhand smoke, 1988–2002. Serum cotinine geometric means and 95% confidence intervals (CIs) in U.S. nonsmokers by study interval. Data are plotted at approximate midpoint for four periods: 1988–1991 (National Health and Nutrition Examination Survey III [NHANES III], phase 1), 1991–1994 (NHANES III, phase 2), 1999–2000, and 2001–2002.
SOURCE: Pirkle et al., 2006.

entire country and include regions with and without smoking regulations, so they reflect the national trend but underestimate the reduction in areas with strong smoke-free regulations (Pirkle et al., 2006).

The effect of voluntary and regulatory smoking bans on exposure of workers can be seen in data from the National Health and Nutrition Examination Survey (NHANES), which show an overall reduction from 1988 to 2002 in serum cotinine concentration in nonsmokers working in the service industry (see Figure 2-3a) (Pickett et al., 2006). Arheart et al. (2008) analyzed serum cotinine concentrations from NHANES data in the same period in workers in different sectors (blue-collar, farm, service industry, and white-collar workers). Serum cotinine concentrations showed a declining trend in all sectors and subgroups analyzed from 1988 to 2002 (Figure 2-3b). Farm workers, who often work outdoors, had the lowest cotinine concentrations initially and the smallest change in those concentrations over time, followed in both respects by white-collar workers. Blue-collar and service-industry workers had higher concentrations initially

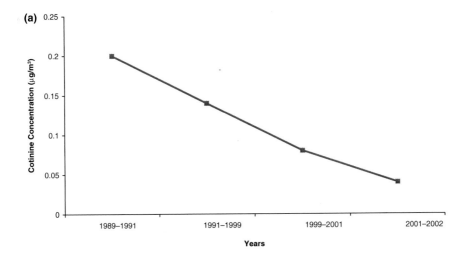

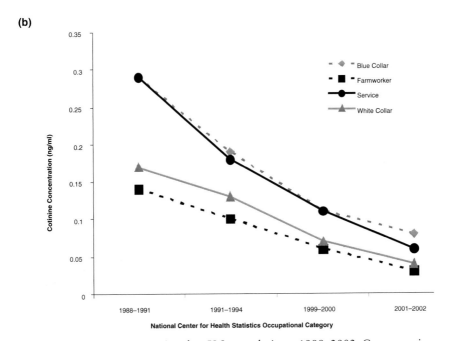

FIGURE 2-3 Serum cotinine in select U.S. populations, 1988–2002. Concentrations were measured in National Health and Nutrition Examination Surveys (NHANES). (a) service workers. Data from Pickett et al., 2006; (b) blue-collar workers, farmworkers, service workers, white-collar workers. Data from Arheart et al., 2008.

and had the greatest declines by 2002. The serum cotinine concentrations in the NHANES data integrate all exposure, including home exposure, and include data from regions where and times when smoking bans were not in place so the reductions in secondhand-smoke exposure when there were smoking bans are much greater than observed here. The reduction in exposure, therefore, could in part reflect voluntary smoking bans in private workplaces, which increased.

Changes in PM, nicotine, and cotinine concentrations after the implementation of smoking bans have been studied. Some of the studies are summarized below.

Airborne Particulate Matter Before and After Smoking Bans

Estimating the contribution of secondhand smoke to airborne PM concentrations requires consideration of background concentrations of respirable particles. Estimates vary widely because of differences in measurement techniques and geographic location. Leaderer and Hammond (1991) have reported PM concentrations in 96 randomly selected residences in New York state: the mean respirable PM in nonsmoking residences was 15 $\mu g/m^3$, compared with 44 $\mu g/m^3$ in smoking homes (average of 71 cigarettes smoked in the homes during the week), which could be considered typical of U.S. residences. The extent to which tobacco smoke contributes to a difference from the background concentration varies greatly. A representative study by Spengler et al. (1981) found that in 35 nonsmoking homes the respirable particle concentration averaged 24 $\mu g/m^3$, while homes with one smoker averaged 36 $\mu g/m^3$ and homes with two smokers averaged 70 $\mu g/m^3$. In recent studies, concentrations of $PM_{2.5}$ in German bars, restaurants, and discotheques where smoking is permitted have been reported to be between 178 and 808 $\mu g/m^3$ measured over 4 hours (Bolte et al., 2008). The particle number concentration was between 120,000 and 210,000 particles per cm^3 and the majority of particles had a size of 0.01–0.5 μm. These results are similar to earlier data obtained from restaurants and bars in Vancouver, British Columbia, which showed a concentration range of 47–253 $\mu g/m^3$ for $PM_{2.5}$ and 51–268 $\mu g/m^3$ for PM_{10} in restaurants with unrestricted smoking measured over 6 hours (Brauer and Mannetje, 1998). A survey of 32 countries found high levels of $PM_{2.5}$ (200–300 $\mu g/m^3$) in countries without a smoking ban (Hyland et al., 2008). Furthermore, significant decreases in PM levels in restaurants have been reported after introduction of smoke-free legislation. In England measurements collected from 49 businesses show a 95% decrease in $PM_{2.5}$ levels from 217 to 11 $\mu g/m^3$ (Gotz et al., 2008). Similar levels of reduction in $PM_{2.5}$ levels of 77% have been reported after implementation of a smoking ban in a North

Carolina correctional facility (Proescholdbell et al., 2008) and of 71–99% in restaurants in Austin, Texas (Waring and Siegel, 2007).

Airborne $PM_{2.5}$ concentrations in restaurants decreased significantly in Ohio, Massachusetts, New York state, Norway, and Italy after the implementation of smoking bans (Akbar-Khanzadeh et al., 2004; Alpert et al., 2007; CDC, 2004, 2007; Ellingsen et al., 2006; Valente et al., 2007). As can be seen in Figure 2-4a, concentrations decreased from 194 to 67 $\mu g/m^3$, from 206 to 14 $\mu g/m^3$, and from 248 to 23.1 $\mu g/m^3$ in Ohio, Massachusetts, and New York state, respectively. Decreases in Norway and Italy were smaller—from 115 to 77 $\mu g/m^3$ and from 110 to 61 $\mu g/m^3$ (CDC, 2004; Ellingsen et al., 2006; Valente et al., 2007)—but initial $PM_{2.5}$ concentrations in European restaurants were lower pre-ban than in the United States. It is important to note that because of the presence of background $PM_{2.5}$, $PM_{2.5}$ concentrations will not reach zero even with 100% compliance with a ban, and most of the concentrations measured after the ban are close to outdoor, or background, concentrations.

Data from New York state, Norway, Scotland, and Italy demonstrated substantial reductions in PM concentrations in other public areas (such as bars and bowling alleys) after implementation of smoking bans (Figure 2-4b). $PM_{2.5}$ concentrations before smoking bans varied widely among studies, from 61 to 549 $\mu g/m^3$ in different indoor settings, but decreased greatly after implementation, to 6 to 40 $\mu g/m^3$ in most venues (background concentrations of $PM_{2.5}$ are typically about 15–30 $\mu g/m^3$). $PM_{2.5}$ decreased, for example, in a study of New York state bars from 549 to about 33 $\mu g/m^3$ (CDC, 2004), in New York state bowling alleys from 61 to about 20 $\mu g/m^3$ [5] (CDC, 2004), and in Scottish pubs from 246 to 20 $\mu g/m^3$ (Semple et al., 2007). Complete smoking bans in the United States, e.g., Massachusetts and New York, led to significant decreases, typically 90%, in $PM_{2.5}$ concentrations to near background levels, except in bars. In Italy and Scotland, post-ban levels in restaurants were half of pre-ban levels and 10–40% of pre-ban levels in other public places.

Airborne Nicotine

Airborne concentrations of nicotine, a tracer that is specific for tobacco smoke, decreased even more dramatically after the implementation of smoking bans. Because there are no other important sources of nicotine, the background airborne concentration of nicotine should be zero.

Data from three countries demonstrated that smoking bans in restaurants led to greater than 90% reductions in airborne nicotine. In Ohio

---

[5] Averages in New York state bars and bowling alleys calculated from the table in CDC (2004).

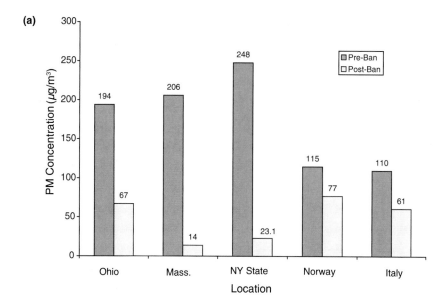

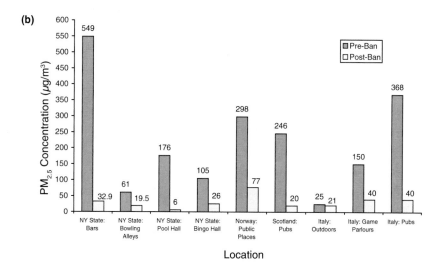

FIGURE 2-4 Airborne PM$_{2.5}$ concentrations in (a) restaurants and (b) public places before and after implementation of smoking bans. Data from Akbar-Khanzadeh et al. (2004) examined exposure in Ohio, which implemented a clean air ordinance allowing smoking in separate sections in restrauants. Data from Akbar-Khanzadeh et al., 2004; Alpert et al., 2007; CDC, 2004; Elligsen et al., 2006; Semple et al., 2007; and Valente et al., 2007.

(Akbar-Khanzadeh et al., 2004), Norway (Ellingsen et al., 2006), and Florence and Belluno, Italy (Gorini et al., 2008), nicotine concentrations in restaurants decreased from 9.8, 28.3, and 2 $\mu g/m^3$, respectively, to less than 0.1 $\mu g/m^3$ after implementation of smoking bans (Figure 2-5a), that is, to less than 5%, and usually <1% pre-ban levels.

Similarly, in other public places (such as pubs and discos), smoking bans resulted in large decreases in airborne nicotine concentrations (Figure 2-5b), from concentrations about 35–165 $\mu g/m^3$ to less than 6 $\mu g/m^3$ after bans were implemented in Norway, Italy, and Ireland (Ellingsen et al., 2006; Gorini et al., 2005, 2008; Mulcahy et al., 2005). For example, Mulcahy et al. (2005) measured the effect of the Irish smoking ban on airborne nicotine concentrations in pubs and cotinine concentrations in hospitality workers. In a sample of 20 bars in Galway, Ireland, air nicotine decreased by 83% (from a median of 36 to 6 $\mu g/m^3$; p < 0.001) between the Friday night preceding the ban and 5 weeks after the ban was implemented (Mulcahy et al., 2005).

In the first multicenter study in Europe, Nebot et al. (2005) measured nicotine vapor concentrations in public places that included transportation, education, and leisure settings (Nebot et al., 2005). The study used passive samplers placed in public places for 4 h to 2 weeks. In cities in seven European countries (in Vienna, Paris, Athens, Florence, Oporto, Barcelona, and Orebro), nicotine concentrations were highest in bars and discos (median 19 $\mu g/m^3$, values up to 122 $\mu g/m^3$), followed by restaurants, airports, and train stations (Nebot et al., 2005). Schools and hospitals had the lowest concentration of nicotine.

In the absence of smoke-free policies, nicotine concentrations in offices can be high. Reduction in workplace exposure to secondhand smoke can have a large effect on overall exposure to secondhand smoke because of the exposure duration of what is typically an 8-h workday in the United States.

Research has compared concentrations of nicotine in workplaces that allowed smoking to those that have policies restricting smoking to a few designated areas and workplaces that have policies that ban smoking in the workplace (see Figure 2-6) (Hammond, 1999). Nicotine concentrations were lower (generally under 1 $\mu g/m^3$) in workplaces that banned smoking than in workplaces that allowed smoking (mean concentrations, generally 2–6 $\mu g/m^3$ in offices, 3–8 $\mu g/m^3$ in restaurants, and 1–6 $\mu g/m^3$ in blue-collar workplaces). Hammond (1999) also reported that workplace concentrations are variable but could be more than 10 times higher than average home concentrations and that for 30% of workers the workplace is the principal source of secondhand smoke (Hammond, 1999).

In a cross-sectional study, sampling at nonsmokers' desks or workstations in 25 Massachusetts office and nonoffice workplaces (such as

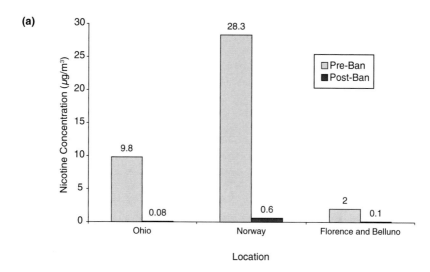

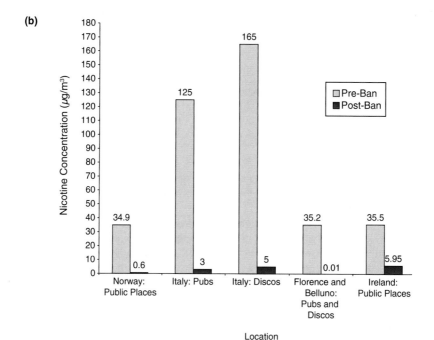

FIGURE 2-5 Airborne nicotine concentrations in (a) restaurants and (b) other public places before and after implementation of smoking bans. Nicotine concentrations represent median not mean amounts in Ireland study. All other data represent mean nicotine concentrations. Data from Akbar-Khanzadeh et al., 2004; Ellingsen et al., 2006; Gorini et al., 2005, 2008; and Mulcahy et al., 2005.

manufacturing, printing workplaces, and fire stations) found that nonoffice workplaces that allowed smoking had nicotine concentrations of 0.1 to over 20 $\mu g/m^3$ (median, 2.3 $\mu g/m^3$). Open offices with several workers had even higher concentrations: a median of 8.6 $\mu g/m^3$ and some values over 40 $\mu g/m^3$ (Figure 2-6a) (Hammond et al., 1995). Those values were markedly different among the companies that did not allow smoking indoors; for nonsmokers, median nonoffice values dropped from 2.3 to 0.2 $\mu g/m^3$ and median values in open offices from 8.6 to 0.3 $\mu g/m^3$ (see Figure 2-6a).

Some research has shown that those who live in homes with smokers who smoke in the home benefit from nonsmoking workplaces. In a reanalysis of the data from the 16 Cities Study (Jenkins et al., 1996)[6] to stratify home smoking status and compare exposures by workplace smoking status, people who were exposed to smoking both at home and at work had over twice the 24-h average exposure compared to those who were exposed in the home but not at work (Barnes et al., 2006). The authors concluded that "if workplaces were smoke-free, the total SHS [secondhand smoke] exposure of those living with smokers could be cut in half, and the total SHS exposure of those living in nonsmoking homes would become negligible, a significant worker safety and public health benefit" (Barnes et al., 2006).

Direct evidence that policies banning smoking in the workplace reduce airborne nicotine can be seen in two studies in which nicotine was measured in offices before and after smoking restrictions were implemented (Vaughan and Hammond, 1990). Vaughan and Hammond (1990) measured nicotine in 30 office locations in one building in Missouri before and after control of secondhand smoke (see Figure 2-6b). Nicotine vapors in the air were measured with passive filters and active pumps. Before the ban, offices with more than one smoker were sometimes shared with nonsmokers. The authors found over a 90% reduction in nicotine concentrations measured at workers' desks after smoking was restricted to the snack bar. Nicotine vapor concentrations decreased in smoker, nonsmoker, and vacant spaces by 81–98% (Vaughan and Hammond, 1990).

A study of 14 office buildings in China evaluated weekly average nicotine concentrations in buildings according to their smoking policies regardless of extent of enforcement (see Figure 2-6b) (Gan et al., 2008). In addition, one building was sampled before and after a smoke-free policy was implemented. The authors found that

---

[6] The 16 Cities Study was originally funded by a tobacco manufacturer. The data used in the study were released as a result of a lawsuit. Jenkins et al. (1996) concluded that the highest exposure of those living with a smoker occurred in the home. The results of the study have been disputed, with analyses of documents from the tobacco industry, a regulatory agency, and court records indicating that the data presented masked the benefits of smoking ban (Barnes and Glantz, 2007).

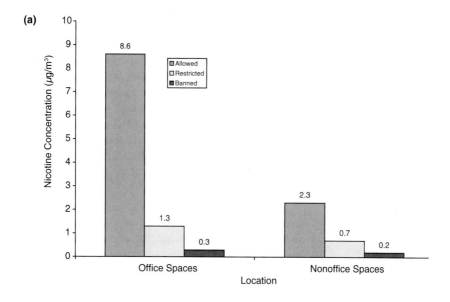

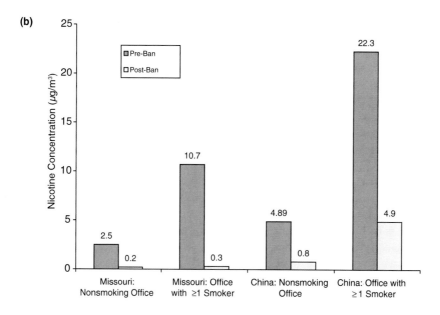

FIGURE 2-6 Occupational exposures to airborne nicotine in (a) a sampling at non-smokers' desks in 25 office and nonoffice workplaces. Data from Hammond et al., 1995; and (b) offices. Data from Gan et al., 2008; Hammond, 1999; and Vaughan and Hammond, 1990.

For all 14 buildings, offices in buildings with smoking policies had less than half SHS as offices without smoking policies. In one building where we sampled the air before and after a smoke-free policy was implemented on January 1, 2006, the SHS concentrations decreased significantly after the policy was enacted.

For example, nicotine concentrations in offices with at least one smoker fell 90% from 18.8 to 1.9 $\mu g/m^3$.

Biomarkers of Secondhand-Smoke Exposure
Before and After Smoking Bans

Evidence indicates that the implementation of smoking bans is effective in reducing individual exposures to secondhand smoke but that exposures do not decrease to zero, because there are other sources of exposure (such as homes and vehicles). Most of the data come from workers in public establishments, such as restaurants, bars, and hotels.

Al-Delaimy et al. (2001) measured nicotine concentrations in the hair of bar and restaurant workers in Wellington and Auckland, New Zealand, when partial smoking restrictions were in place that required restaurants to designate 50% of seating as smoke-free and bars were exempt from restrictions. In nonsmokers, hair nicotine varied with the type of smoke-free policy in the workplace, which was categorized as 100% smoke-free, 50% smoke-free, or no restrictions. People working in smoke-free establishments had significantly lower hair nicotine concentrations (0.62 ng/mg; Kruskal-Wallis $\chi^2 = 26.4$; $p < 0.0001$) than people in 50% smoke-free establishments (2.72 ng/mg) or establishments with no restrictions (6.69 ng/mg).

In Norway, Ellingsen et al. (2006) showed decreased exposure to secondhand smoke, as demonstrated by decreased cotinine concentrations, in the urine of nonsmoking employees of restaurants and bars and decreased air concentrations of nicotine and decreased total dust concentrations in the 13 establishments surveyed after the implementation of a ban on smoking in bars and restaurants.

Data on employees of public establishments in New York state (Farrelly et al., 1999), Scotland (Menzies et al., 2006), Ireland (Mulcahy et al., 2005), and Italy (Valente et al., 2007) demonstrate large decreases in exposure after implementation of smoking bans (see Figure 2-7a). In the New York state study, saliva cotinine concentrations decreased from 3.6 to 0.78 ng/mL; in Scotland, serum cotinine concentrations decreased from 5.15 to 2.93 ng/mL; in Ireland, salivary cotinine concentrations decreased from 2.86 to 1.29 ng/mL; and in Italy, urinary cotinine concentrations decreased from 17.8 to 5.5 ng/mL. In Ireland (Mulcahy et al., 2005), data were categorized by type of staff in hotels (Figure 2-7b): waiters had the largest

(a)

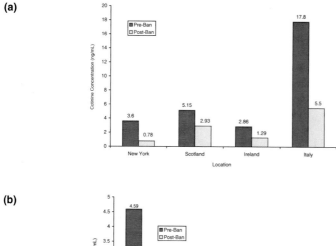

(b)

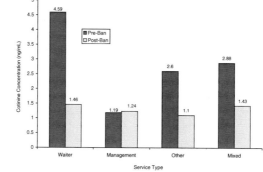

(C)

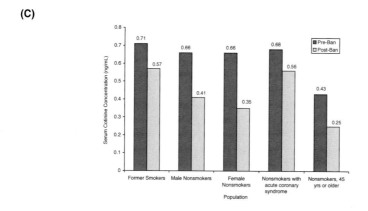

FIGURE 2-7 Exposures to secondhand smoke in (a) workers in public establishments, (b) hotel staff in Ireland, and (c) former smokers and nonsmokers in Scotland. Data from New York state and Ireland are salivary cotinine concentrations. Data from Scotland are serum cotinine concentrations. Data from Italy are urinary cotinine concentrations. Data from Farrelly et al., 2005; Menzies et al., 2006; Mulcahy et al., 2005; Pell et al., 2008; and Valente et al., 2007.

decrease in salivary cotinine, from 4.59 to 1.46 ng/mL, and management had a low cotinine concentration both before and after the ban (1.19 and 1.24 ng/mL, respectively).

Pell et al. (2008) showed reductions in serum cotinine concentrations in a variety of demographic groups after implementation of the Scottish smoking ban, including former smokers, male and female nonsmokers, nonsmokers with acute coronary syndrome, and nonsmokers over 45 years old (Figure 2-7c) (Pell et al., 2008). The largest decreases occurred in nonsmokers.

Pickett et al. (2006) used data from the NHANES surveys to examine the relationship between smoke-free laws and secondhand-smoke exposure of nonsmoking adults in the United States. The authors categorized 57 NHANES locations as to their smoke-free law coverage ("extensive," "limited," or "no laws") and looked at serum cotinine concentrations in nonsmokers, as defined by self-reported smoking status and serum cotinine concentrations (a concentration below 10 ng/mL was considered that of a nonsmoker). Both male and female nonsmokers living in areas with extensive smoke-free laws had significantly lower probabilities of having detectable cotinine (at least 0.05 ng/mL) than those who lived in areas without smoke-free laws. For example, the percentage of nonsmoking men with detectable cotinine dropped from 57% in areas with only limited restriction to only 10% in areas with extensive smoke-free regulations; for women, the decline was from 90% to 19%.

CONCLUSIONS

- Airborne tracers of secondhand smoke and biomarkers of exposure to secondhand smoke are complementary. Airborne tracers measure concentrations in specific venues while biomarkers integrate all sources of exposure and incorporate inhalation rates. Because of its short half-life, cotinine reflects only recent exposures. NNAL has a longer half-life, but has not been used as widely. Concentrations of cotinine in serum, saliva, and urine are specific indicators of total exposure to secondhand smoke. Airborne measures of exposure can demonstrate the contribution of different sources or venues of exposure but do not reflect total dose unless all venues are measured.
- The concentration of airborne nicotine is a specific tracer for secondhand smoke. PM can also be used as an indication of secondhand-smoke exposure but, because there are other sources of PM, it is a less specific tracer than nicotine.
- Both airborne monitoring studies and biomonitoring studies demonstrate that exposure to secondhand smoke is substantially re-

duced after implementation of smoking bans. Air concentrations of nicotine and PM decreased by more than 80% in restaurants, bars, and workplaces in most studies after smoking bans were implemented; serum and salivary cotinine concentrations decreased by 50% or more in most studies. The residual concentration reflects continued exposure in unregulated areas, such as homes.

REFERENCES

Akbar-Khanzadeh, F., S. Milz, A. Ames, S. Spino, and C. Tex. 2004. Effectiveness of clean indoor air ordinances in controlling environmental tobacco smoke in restaurants. *Archives of Environmental Health* 59(12):677-685.

Al-Delaimy, W., T. Fraser, and A. Woodward. 2001. Nicotine in hair of bar and restaurant workers. *New Zealand Medical Journal* 114(1127):80-83.

Alpert, H. R., C. M. Carpenter, M. J. Travers, and G. N. Connolly. 2007. Environmental and economic evaluation of the Massachusetts smoke-free workplace law. *Journal of Community Health* 32(4):269-281.

Arheart, K. L., D. J. Lee, N. A. Dietz, J. D. Wilkinson, J. D. Clark, 3rd, W. G. LeBlanc, B. Serdar, and L. E. Fleming. 2008. Declining trends in serum cotinine levels in US worker groups: The power of policy. *Journal of Occupational & Environmental Medicine* 50(1):57-63.

Barnes, R. L., and S. A. Glantz. 2007. Endotoxins in tobacco smoke: Shifting tobacco industry positions. *Nicotine and Tobacco Research* 9(10):995-1004.

Barnes, R. L., S. K. Hammond, and S. A. Glantz. 2006. The tobacco industry's role in the 16 Cities Study of secondhand tobacco smoke: Do the data support the stated conclusions? *Environmental Health Perspectives* 114(12):1890-1897.

Benner, C., J. M. Bayona, F. M. Caka, H. Tang, L. Lewis, J. Crawford, J. Lamb, M. I. Lee, E. A. Lewis, L. D. Hansen, and D. J. Eatough. 1989. Chemical composition of environmental tobacco smoke. 2. Particulate phase compounds. *Environmental Science Technology* 23:688-699.

Benowitz, N. L. 1999. The biology of nicotine dependence: From the 1988 surgeon general's report to the present and into the future. *Nicotine & Tobacco Research* 1 Suppl 2: S159-S163.

Benowitz, N. L., J. T. Bernert, R. S. Caraballo, D. B. Holiday, and J. Wang. 2009. Optimal serum cotinine levels for distinguishing cigarette smokers and nonsmokers within different racial/ethnic groups in the United States between 1999 and 2004. *American Journal of Epidemiology* 169(2):236-248.

Bolte, G., D. Heitmann, M. Kiranoglu, R. Schierl, J. Diemer, W. Koerner, and H. Fromme. 2008. Exposure to environmental tobacco smoke in German restaurants, pubs and discotheques. *Journal of Exposure Science & Environmental Epidemiology* 18(3):262-271.

Brauer, M., and A. Mannetje. 1998. Restaurant smoking restrictions and environmental tobacco smoke exposure. *American Journal of Public Health* 88(12):1834-1836.

Cal EPA (California Environmental Protection Agency). 2005a. *Proposed identification of environmental tobacco smoke as a toxic air contaminant. Part A: Exposure assessment.* Sacramento: California Environmental Protection Agency.

———. 2005b. *Proposed identification of environmental tobacco smoke as a toxic air contaminant. Part B: Health effects.* Sacramento: California Environmental Protection Agency.

CDC (Centers for Disease Control and Prevention). 2004. Indoor air quality in hospitality venues before and after implementation of a clean indoor air law—western New York, 2003. MMWR—Morbidity & Mortality Weekly Report 53(44):1038-1041.

———. 2006. Fact sheet: Secondhand smoke. (Accessed December 2008, from http://www. cdc.gov/tobacco/data_statistics/fact_sheets/secondhand_smoke/secondhandsmoke.htm).

———. 2007. Reduced secondhand smoke exposure after implementation of a comprehensive statewide smoking ban—New York, June 26, 2003-June 30, 2004. MMWR—Morbidity & Mortality Weekly Report 56(28):705-708.

Daisey, J. M. 1999. Tracers for assessing exposure to environmental tobacco smoke: What are they tracing? Environmental Health Perspectives 107 Suppl 2:319-327.

Eatough, D., C. Benner, J. Bayona, G. Richards, J. Lamb, M. Lee, E. Lewis, and L. Hansen. 1989. Chemical composition of environmental tobacco smoke. 1. Gas-phase acids and bases. Environmental Science Technology 23(6):679-687.

Ellingsen, D. G., G. Fladseth, H. L. Daae, M. Gjolstad, K. Kjaerheim, M. Skogstad, R. Olsen, S. Thorud, and P. Molander. 2006. Airborne exposure and biological monitoring of bar and restaurant workers before and after the introduction of a smoking ban. Journal of Environmental Monitoring 8(3):362-368.

Emmons, K. M., S. K. Hammond, J. L. Fava, W. F. Velicer, J. L. Evans, and A. D. Monroe. 2001. A randomized trial to reduce passive smoke exposure in low-income households with young children. Pediatrics 108(1):18-24.

Farrelly, M. C., W. N. Evans, and A. E. Sfekas. 1999. The impact of workplace smoking bans: Results from a national survey. Tobacco Control 8(3):272-277.

Gan, Q., S. K. Hammond, Y. Jiang, Y. Yang, and T. W. Hu. 2008. Effectiveness of a smoke-free policy in lowering secondhand smoke concentrations in offices in China. Journal of Occupational & Environmental Medicine 50(5):570-575.

Gorini, G., A. Gasparrini, M. C. Fondelli, A. S. Costantini, F. Centrich, M. J. Lopez, M. Nebot, and E. Tamang. 2005. Environmental tobacco smoke (ETS) exposure in Florence hospitality venues before and after the smoking ban in Italy. Journal of Occupational & Environmental Medicine 47(12):1208-1210; author reply 1210.

Gorini, G., H. Moshammer, L. Sbrogio, A. Gasparrini, M. Nebot, M. Neuberger, E. Tamang, M. J. Lopez, D. Galeone, and E. Serrahima. 2008. Italy and Austria Before and After study: Second-hand smoke exposure in hospitality premises before and after 2 years from the introduction of the Italian smoking ban. Indoor Air 18(4):328-334.

Gotz, N. K., M. van Tongeren, H. Wareing, L. M. Wallace, S. Semple, and L. Maccalman. 2008. Changes in air quality and second-hand smoke exposure in hospitality sector businesses after introduction of the English smoke-free legislation. Journal of Public Health (Oxford, England) 30(4):421-428.

Hammond, S. K. 1999. Exposure of U.S. workers to environmental tobacco smoke. Environmental Health Perspectives 107 Suppl 2:329-340.

Hammond, S. K., J. Coghlin, P. H. Gann, M. Paul, K. Taghizadeh, P. L. Skipper, and S. R. Tannenbaum. 1993. Relationship between environmental tobacco smoke exposure and carcinogen-hemoglobin adduct levels in nonsmokers. Journal of the National Cancer Institute 85(6):474-478.

Hammond, S. K., G. Sorensen, R. Youngstrom, and J. K. Ockene. 1995. Occupational exposure to environmental tobacco smoke. JAMA 274(12):956-960.

Hecht, S. S. 2004. Carcinogen derived biomarkers: Applications in studies of human exposure to secondhand tobacco smoke. Tobacco Control 13 Suppl 1:i48-i56.

Hinds, W. C. 1999. Aerosol technology: Properties, behavior, and measurement of airborne particles. 2nd ed. New York: John Wiley & Sons, Inc.

Hukkanen, J., P. Jacob, 3rd, and N. L. Benowitz. 2005. Metabolism and disposition kinetics of nicotine. Pharmacological Review 57(1):79-115.

Hyland, A., M. J. Travers, C. Dresler, C. Higbee, and K. M. Cummings. 2008. A 32-country comparison of tobacco smoke derived particle levels in indoor public places. *Tobacco Control* 17(3):159-165.

Jenkins, R. A., A. Palausky, R. W. Counts, C. K. Bayne, A. B. Dindal, and M. R. Guerin. 1996. Exposure to environmental tobacco smoke in sixteen cities in the United States as determined by personal breathing zone air sampling. *Journal of Exposure Analysis and Environmental Epidemiology* 6(4):473-502.

Jenkins, R., M. R. Guerin, and B. A. Tomkins. 2000. *The chemistry of environmental tobacco smoke: Composition and measurement.* Boca Raton, FL: Lewis Publishers.

Kraev, T. A., G. Adamkiewicz, S. K. Hammond, and J. D. Spengler. 2009. Indoor concentrations of nicotine in low-income, multi-family housing: Associations with smoking behaviors and housing characteristics. *Tobacco Control* 18(6):438-444.

Kritz, H., P. Schmid, and H. Sinzinger. 1995. Passive smoking and cardiovascular risk. *Archives of Internal Medicine* 155(18):1942-1948.

Leaderer, B. P., and S. K. Hammond. 1991. Evaluation of vapor-phase nicotine and respirable suspended particle mass as markers for environmental tobacco smoke. *Environmental Science and Technology* 25(4):770-777.

Lodovici, M., V. Akpan, C. Evangelisti, and P. Dolara. 2004. Sidestream tobacco smoke as the main predictor of exposure to polycyclic aromatic hydrocarbons. *Journal of Applied Toxicology* 24(4):277-281.

Menzies, D., A. Nair, P. A. Williamson, S. Schembri, M. Z. H. Al-Khairalla, M. Barnes, T. C. Fardon, L. McFarlane, G. J. Magee, and B. J. Lipworth. 2006. Respiratory symptoms, pulmonary function, and markers of inflammation among bar workers before and after a legislative ban on smoking in public places. *JAMA* 296(14):1742-1748.

Mulcahy, M., D. S. Evans, S. K. Hammond, J. L. Repace, and M. Byrne. 2005. Secondhand smoke exposure and risk following the Irish smoking ban: An assessment of salivary cotinine concentrations in hotel workers and air nicotine levels in bars. *Tobacco Control* 14(6):384-388.

Nebot, M., M. J. Lopez, G. Gorini, M. Neuberger, S. Axelsson, M. Pilali, C. Fonseca, K. Abdennbi, A. Hackshaw, H. Moshammer, A. M. Laurent, J. Salles, M. Georgouli, M. C. Fondelli, E. Serrahima, F. Centrich, and S. K. Hammond. 2005. Environmental tobacco smoke exposure in public places of European cities. *Tobacco Control* 14(1):60-63.

NRC (National Research Council). 1986. *Environmental tobacco smoke: Measuring exposures and assessing health effects.* Washington, DC: National Academy Press.

———. 2006. *Human biomonitoring for environmental chemicals.* Washington, DC: The National Academies Press.

Pell, J. P., S. Haw, S. Cobbe, D. E. Newby, A. C. H. Pell, C. Fischbacher, A. McConnachie, S. Pringle, D. Murdoch, F. Dunn, K. Oldroyd, P. Macintyre, B. O'Rourke, and W. Borland. 2008. Smoke-free legislation and hospitalizations for acute coronary syndrome. *New England Journal of Medicine* 359(5):482-491.

Pickett, M. S., S. E. Schober, D. J. Brody, L. R. Curtin, and G. A. Giovino. 2006. Smoke-free laws and secondhand smoke exposure in US non-smoking adults, 1999-2002. *Tobacco Control* 15(4):302-307.

Pirkle, J. L., J. T. Bernert, S. P. Caudill, C. S. Sosnoff, and T. F. Pechacek. 2006. Trends in the exposure of nonsmokers in the U.S. population to secondhand smoke: 1988-2002. *Environmental Health Perspectives* 114(6):853-858.

Proescholdbell, S. K., K. L. Foley, J. Johnson, and S. H. Malek. 2008. Indoor air quality in prisons before and after implementation of a smoking ban law. *Tobacco Control* 17(2):123-127.

Schick, S., and S. Glantz. 2005. Philip Morris toxicological experiments with fresh sidestream smoke: More toxic than mainstream smoke. *Tobacco Control* 14(6):396-404.

Schick, S., and S. A. Glantz. 2006. Sidestream cigarette smoke toxicity increases with aging and exposure duration. *Tobacco Control* 15(6):424-429.

Schick, S. F., and S. Glantz. 2007. Concentrations of the carcinogen 4-(methylnitrosamino)-1-(3-pyridyl)-1-butanone in sidestream cigarette smoke increase after release into indoor air: Results from unpublished tobacco industry research. *Cancer Epidemiology, Biomarkers & Prevention* 16(8):1547-1553.

Semple, S., K. S. Creely, A. Naji, B. G. Miller, and J. G. Ayres. 2007. Secondhand smoke levels in Scottish pubs: The effect of smoke-free legislation. *Tobacco Control* 16(2):127-132.

Singer, B. C., A. T. Hodgson, K. S. Guevarra, E. L. Hawley, and W. W. Nazaroff. 2002. Gas-phase organics in environmental tobacco smoke. 1. Effects of smoking rate, ventilation, and furnishing level on emission factors. *Environmental Science Technology* 36(5):846-853.

Spengler, J. D., D. W. Dockery, W. A. Turner, J. M. Wolfson, and B. G. Ferris Jr. 1981. Long-term measurements of respirable particulates and implications for air pollution epidemiology. *Atmospheric Environment* 15:23-30.

Valente, P., F. Forastiere, A. Bacosi, G. Cattani, S. Di Carlo, M. Ferri, I. Figa-Talamanca, A. Marconi, L. Paoletti, C. Perucci, and P. Zuccaro. 2007. Exposure to fine and ultrafine particles from secondhand smoke in public places before and after the smoking ban, Italy 2005. *Tobacco Control* 16(5):312-317.

Van Deusen, A., A. Hyland, M. J. Travers, C. Wang, C. Higbee, B. A. King, T. Alford, and K. M. Cummings. 2009. Secondhand smoke and particulate matter exposure in the home. *Nicotine & Tobacco Research* 11(6):635-641.

Vaughan, W. M., and S. K. Hammond. 1990. Impact of "designated smoking area" policy on nicotine vapor and particle concentrations in a modern office building. *Journal of the Air & Waste Management Association* 40(7):1012-1017.

Wamboldt, F. S., R. C. Balkissoon, A. E. Rankin, S. J. Szefler, S. K. Hammond, R. E. Glasgow, and W. P. Dickinson. 2008. Correlates of household smoking bans in low-income families of children with and without asthma. *Fam Process* 47(1):81-94.

Waring, M. S., and J. A. Siegel. 2007. An evaluation of the indoor air quality in bars before and after a smoking ban in Austin, Texas. *Journal of Exposure Science & Environmental Epidemiology* 17(3):260-268.

3

Experimental Studies Relevant to the Pathophysiology of Secondhand Smoke

This chapter discusses pathophysiologic experiments that have investigated the cardiovascular effects of mainstream and sidestream tobacco smoke in cells, in animals, and in humans. It addresses the association between secondhand-smoke exposure and acute coronary events. Specifically it provides information on the biological plausibility of a causal relationship between secondhand smoke exposure and acute coronary events (Question 2, see Box 1-1) and information on the duration of exposure and time following cessation of exposure within which effects might be observed (Questions 3 and 5, see Box 1-1).

The studies reviewed include those with exposure to secondhand smoke and exposure to specific constituents of secondhand smoke. When secondhand smoke was used, the studies were conducted with cigarette smoke, not smoke from cigars, pipes, or hookahs. Typically, reference cigarettes (cigarettes that are manufactured according to a standard formula for research purposes to provide researchers a consistent and uniform test item) or Marlboro cigarettes are used. Studies have not demonstrated much variation in constituents among cigarette brands and types (HHS, 2001), nor in the concentrations of constituents in secondhand smoke (Daisey, 1999).

As discussed by Hatsukami et al. (2006), "several physiological changes involving potential mechanisms of smoking-induced cardiovascular disease have been observed in cigarette smokers compared with nonsmokers" who have not been exposed to secondhand smoke.

Cigarette smoke, either mainstream or secondhand smoke, could produce cardiovascular disease by a number of interrelated modes of action, including oxidative stress, hemodyamic and autonomic effects, endothelial

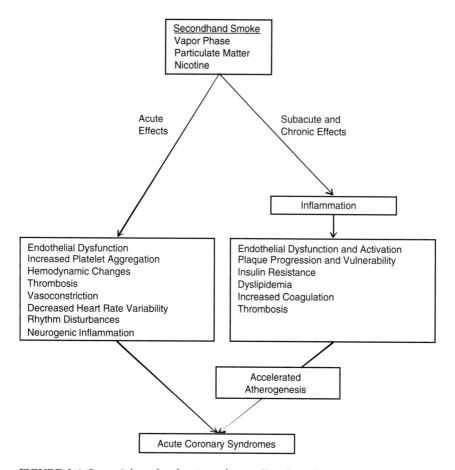

FIGURE 3-1 Potential mode of action of secondhand smoke.
NOTE: Schematic showing cardiovascular effects of secondhand smoke and how they might lead to acute myocardial infarction.

dysfunction, thrombosis, inflammation, hyperlipidemia or other effects (see Figure 3-1). Evidence related to those potential actions is discussed below, followed by a discussion of the effects of the individual constituents of secondhand smoke. Although those physiological changes have been observed and used to assess possible modes of action of secondhand smoke, to date most have not been formally validated as clinical tests and there is not a consensus within the scientific community that they are predictive of actual clinical disease (Ledford, 2008; Wang, 2008; WHO, 2007). Furthermore, a lack of specificity of exposure to secondhand smoke for those markers precludes their use as biomarkers that indicate a given case of cardiovascular disease is caused by exposure to secondhand smoke (Hatsukami et al., 2006). In this section, however, the committee uses those effects to examine whether secondhand-smoke exposure causes pathophysiologic changes that would contribute to the biological plausibility that decreasing secondhand-smoke exposure could lead to a decrease in acute myocardial infarctions (MIs).

EFFECTS OF CIGARETTE SMOKE

Oxidative Stress

As discussed in several review articles (for examples, see Armani et al., 2009; Burke and FitzGerald, 2003), oxidative stress could mediate many of the effects of smoke on the cardiovascular system. Such stress, during which endogenous antioxidants are overwhelmed by oxidants such as reactive oxygen species and free radicals, results in impaired cellular function. The exact mechanisms whereby oxidative stress leads to cardiovascular disease, such as atherosclerosis, are not clear, but it appears that oxidative stress may play a role in cardiovascular pathophysiology (Ballinger et al., 2002), and it could account for many effects of tobacco-smoke exposure, such as endothelial dysfunction, thrombosis, and inflammation (Raupach et al., 2006; Thomas et al., 2008).

Many constituents of mainstream and sidestream smoke are or produce free radicals capable of producing oxidative stress. Those constituents include vapor-phase carbonyl compounds (such as acrolein), oxides of nitrogen, metabolites of polycyclic aromatic hydrocarbons (PAHs), metals, and particulate matter (PM) (NRC, 1986). Mainstream cigarette smoke increases the concentrations of markers of oxidative stress, lipid peroxidation, protein oxidation, and DNA modification. Isoprostanes, indicators of lipid peroxidation and in vivo oxidation injury, are higher in smokers than in nonsmokers, and their concentrations decreased after smoking cessation for 2 weeks (Morrow et al., 1995). Smokers admitted to a cardiac outpatient center who then quit smoking had decreases in isoprostanes a few days after quitting, and the decreases continued until a steady state was reached 4 weeks after quiting (Pilz et al., 2000). Pignatelli et al. (2001) demonstrated that oxidized plasma proteins, another marker of oxidative stress, are higher in smokers than in nonsmokers.

Ahmadzadehfar et al. (2006) reported that exposure to secondhand smoke significantly increased isoprostane 8-epi-PGF$_{2\alpha}$ in nonsmokers. After repeated secondhand-smoke exposure, isoprostane 8-epi-PGF$_{2\alpha}$ in nonsmokers reached nearly the same values as in smokers.

Probst-Hensch (2008) investigated whether the effects of secondhand smoke on the cardiovascular system are mediated by oxidative stress in a sample of 1,122 nonsmoking subjects enrolled in an air-pollution study. Secondhand-smoke exposure was measured based on self-report during an interview as to "how many hours per day they were exposed to other people's tobacco smoke (a) at home, (b) at the workplace, (c) in bars and restaurants, and (d) elsewhere." Exposures were categorized as less than or equal to two hours per day, or more than two hours per day. The role of oxidative stress was assessed by looking at the interactions between glutathione S-transferase (GST) deficiency, which exhibits antioxidative properties, and the effects of secondhand smoke exposure on heart rate variability (HRV), a measure reflecting autonomic cardiac function. HRV was assessed from a 24-hour electrocardiogram recording, and subjects were genotyped for GSTM1, GSTT1, and GSTP1, GSTM1, GSTT1, and GSTP1 polymorphisms interacted with secondhand-smoke exposure to affect HRV. For example, the decrease in HRV in people exposed to secondhand smoke for more than two hours per day was greater when the GSTM1 genotype was deleted as compared to not deleted. That suggests a role of oxidative stress in secondhand smoke's effects on HRV.

Furthermore, animal data reviewed in the surgeon general's report (HHS, 2006) indicate that exposure to secondhand smoke worsens ischemic heart-event outcomes through free-radical activity. Animal data showed that a 30-min exposure to secondhand smoke resulted in oxidative DNA damage in the myocardium as measured by increases in 8-hydroxydeoxyguanosine. Secondhand-smoke exposure also activates neutrophils, which leads to oxidation and tissue damage.

Data in animals also show oxidative effects. Secondhand-smoke exposure (30 mg/m^3 total suspended particles from cigarette smoke, or equivalent to about two cigarettes every 15 minutes, for 6 hours per day, 5 days per week for 3 or 8 weeks) increased mitochondrial DNA damage in aortic tissue, which can be caused by increased reactive oxygen and nitrogen species, of apoE -/- mice (mice that lack a high-affinity ligand for lipoprotein receptors that result in them developing atherosclerotic plaques similar to those in humans) (Knight-Lozano et al., 2002). Data on apoE -/- mouse and human tissue indicate that mitochondrial DNA damage might be an early event in atherosclerosis (Ballinger et al., 2002). Eaton et al. (2006) examined the effect of acute tobacco-smoke exposure on mitochondrial function and calcium handling of cardiac cells in rats. Mitochondria were isolated after 6 h of secondhand smoke exposure (about 60 mg/m^3, with an average nicotine concentration of 6.95 ± 0.62 mg/m^3). Mitochondria from smoke-exposed rats had significantly higher adenosine diphosphate–stimulated production of adenosine triphosphate, had a more reduced redox state (nicotinamide adenine dinucleotide [NADH] ratio), showed more rapid membrane depolarization in response to calcium, and had significantly increased cyclosporin A–sensitive Ca^{2+} release, although net Ca^{2+} uptake was unchanged.

Autonomic Effects

Cigarette smoke could affect the cardiovascular system through the autonomic nervous system, associated hemodynamic effects, or both. Heart rate is regulated by the interaction between the sympathetic and parasympathetic nervous systems. Sympathetic nervous system activation reduces heart-rate variability, and decreased heart-rate variability is associated with higher risk of cardiac death and of arrhythmic events after an acute MI (Buccelletti et al., 2009).

Smoking can have direct effects on heart rate, and those effects are thought to be mediated by actions on the sympathetic component of the autonomic nervous system. Nicotine acts on nicotinic cholinergic receptors in the brain and adrenal glands to activate the sympathetic nervous system, and this leads to epinephrine release. Nicotine thus acts as a sympathomimetic drug in increasing heart rate, blood pressure, and cardiac contractility and constricting some blood vessels (Haass and Kubler, 1997). Studies show that cigarette smoking increases a person's heart rate (Benowitz et al., 1984; Minami et al., 1999). In the study by Minami et al. (1999) heart rate was higher by an average of 7 beats per minute while smoking compared to when not smoking, and smoking cessation for a week decreased heart rate.

Although nicotine from cigarette smoke transiently increases blood pressure, cigarette smoke has not been associated with hypertension in epidemiologic studies (HHS, 2004). Nicotine constricts coronary arteries via alpha-adrenergic effects (Winniford et al., 1986), and the coronary vasoconstriction is greater in diseased than in healthy coronary arteries (Nicod et al., 1984). In healthy smokers, coronary blood flow (CBF) increases in response to the cigarette smoking- or nicotine-mediated increase in myocardial work. In the absence of nicotine, however, the magnitude of the increase in myocardial work is less in healthy smokers. In people with coronary arterial disease, nicotine and cigarette smoke decrease CBF. Cigarette smoking is a strong risk factor for coronary vasospasm and for inadequacy of response to vasodilator medication (Caralis et al., 1992).

Secondhand smoke has been shown to affect heart-rate variability. Dietrich et al. (2007) examined the relationship between exposure to secondhand smoke and reduction in heart-rate variability. The study examined 1,218 nonsmokers ages 50 years and older who were participating in the Swiss Cohort Study on Air Pollution and Lung Disease in Adults (SAPALDIA) in 2001–2003. Those exposed to secondhand smoke for more than 2 h/day had lower heart-rate variability and a 2.7% higher heart rate

(95% CI, –0.01 to 5.34%) than those not exposed. The effects of second-hand smoke on heart-rate variability are similar to those observed after exposure to PM (Dietrich et al., 2007).

Argacha et al. (2008) further examined the vascular effects of second-hand smoke exposure to assess whether the effects are mediated by a non-specific reaction to smoke, or are more unique to tobacco smoke, the role of nicotine in the effects, the persistence of the effects following cessation of exposure, and the effect of secondhand smoke on microvascular function measured by skin blood flow. Using a cross-over design, the researchers exposed 11 healthy men to secondhand smoke, smoke from herbal cigarettes, or air (1 h exposure using a hermetic, 1-m^3 Plexiglass box over the head of the subject, with a total of 6 cigarettes lit one every 10 minutes). Heart rate and aortic wave reflection increased and transit time decreased following exposure to secondhand-tobacco smoke, but not smoke from herbal cigarettes or air. None of the exposures affected blood pressure. Skin blood flow at normal temperature was unchanged by any of the treatments but was decreased in response to heating after exposure to secondhand-tobacco smoke. None of the effects of secondhand smoke persisted 20 minutes after exposure. A separate group of 14 men received 2 mg nicotine via a sublingual tablet; in those subjects, the effects on aortic wave reflection were related to the serum nicotine concentrations, indicating a possible role of nicotine in these effects seen after exposure to secondhand smoke.

Endothelial Dysfunction

The vascular endothelium, which lines the arteries, is a semipermeable layer of cells that are involved in the modulation of platelet activation, leukocyte adhesion, thrombosis, and regulation of vascular tone. It plays an important role in the regulation of blood flow, controlling the dilation and constriction of arteries (Hadi et al., 2005). Part of that regulation is through the production of vasoactive substances by the endothelial cells, including nitric oxide (NO), endothelin, prostacyclin, and angiotensinogen (Al-Qaisi et al., 2008). Endothelial dysfunction is one of the key early steps in the pathway to atherosclerosis (Hadi et al., 2005).

Oxidant chemicals produce endothelial dysfunction both by injuring endothelial cells and by degrading NO, the latter of which normally has vasodilator and antiplatelet activity (Heiss et al., 2008; Zhang et al., 2006). Impaired endothelial function in smokers, as measured by flow-mediated dilation of the brachial artery, can be reversed, at least in part, by antioxidants (de Sousa et al., 2005; Neunteufl et al., 2000; Raitakari et al., 2000; Takase et al., 2004; Young et al., 2006). Nicotine was also reported to impair endothelial function acutely in human smokers. Smokers also have increased markers of endothelial dysfunction (Rocchi et al., 2007).

As discussed in the surgeon general's report on secondhand smoke (HHS, 2006), data from experiments in animals and humans demonstrate that secondhand smoke also disrupts endothelial function by reducing NO. Endothelium-dependent vasodilation in nonsmokers is affected by chronic and acute exposures to secondhand smoke.

Mack et al. (2003) examined the effect of chronic exposure to secondhand smoke on arterial wall stiffness in baseline data from 227 never smokers (102 men, 125 women) enrolled in a clinical trial looking at Vitamin E treatment. Ultrasound images were used to measure arterial diameter and carotid artery intima-media thickness (IMT). A carotid stiffness index beta, computed using the change in arterial diameter between maximum and minimum dilation, was used as an indicator of arterial wall stiffness. Smoking and secondhand-smoke exposures (number of smokers and hours per day exposed at home, number of daily exposures at work and outside the home and work) were ascertained through a questionnaire. The stiffness index was associated with body mass index, fasting glucose, and IMT. The stiffness index was not related to exposure to secondhand smoke in the overall study population, but did increase with increased number and daily sources of exposure to secondhand smoke in those subjects with a body mass index of 27.1 kg/m^2 or higher, ages 55 years or older, or with an IMT of 0.707 mm or higher. No other associations were statistically significant, including separate analyses by sex and age.

Heiss et al. (2008) exposed healthy nonsmokers to smoke-free air or secondhand smoke for 30 min on two nonconsecutive days and measured markers of endothelial dysfunction (Heiss et al., 2008). Plasma cotinine concentrations were unchanged after exposure to smoke-free air and reached about 0.3 ng/mL, a level "commonly observed in passive smokers" after exposure to secondhand smoke. The secondhand-smoke exposure increased endothelial progenitor cells (EPCs) and plasma vascular endothelial growth factor but eliminated EPC chemotaxis and decreased endothelial function as measured by flow-mediated dilation (FMD). The effects on FMD returned to normal after 2.5 h, but the effects on endothelial growth factors were still increased after 24 h. The detection of endothelial-cell damage in the blood as a result of short-term exposure to secondhand smoke suggests endothelial damage.

A 30-min exposure to secondhand smoke in a smoking room significantly reduced the coronary flow-velocity reserve in nonsmokers to a level similar to that seen in smokers before and after exposure to secondhand smoke (Otsuka et al., 2001). A 5-min exposure to secondhand smoke (mean carbon monoxide level in the exposure chamber, 30 parts per million) significantly reduced aortic distensibility in nonsmokers and smokers (Stefanadis et al., 1998).

Arterial stiffness can result in the impairment of the elasticity of the aorta. Mahmud and Feely (2004) used wave reflection in the aorta as a marker of arterial stiffness to study the effect of exposure to secondhand smoke (15 cigarettes lit in an unventilated room over the course of 1 hour) on healthy nonsmokers (10 men, 11 women). No baseline differences were seen between the controls and treated groups. Following exposure to secondhand smoke brachial and aortic systolic blood pressure increased in males but not females, and an abnormality was observed in the radial and aortic pressure waveforms; no changes were seen in brachial or aortic diastolic blood pressure, heart rate, or left ventricular ejection duration in either sex. No changes were seen in a control group (6 men, 6 women) exposed to air only.

Kato et al. (2006) examined FMD in the bronchial artery and 8-iso-prostane levels as indicators of vascular endothelial function and oxidative stress, respectively, in 30 male subjects (15 smokers who had abstained from smoking for at least 12 hours, 15 nonsmokers) exposed to secondhand smoke from 15 cigarettes (in a room 3 meters by 4 meters with a 2.5 meter ceiling with ventilation) for 30 minutes. FMD was lower and the levels of 8-isoprostane were higher at baseline in smokers than nonsmokers; neither changed in smokers. In nonsmokers, however, FMD decreased and the levels of 8-isoprostane increased following exposure to secondhand smoke.

Giannini et al. (2007) studied the effects of exposure to secondhand smoke (20 minutes in a 60 cubic meter enclosed space with 15 to 20 cigarettes smoked, achieving 30–35 ppm carbon monoxide) on vascular reactivity of the brachial artery (measured by FMD) in 18 healthy, nonsmoking volunteers. Carboxyhemaglobin was elevated after exposure to secondhand smoke. FMD was decreased following the exposure, but nitroglycerin-induced vasodilation was not changed significantly.

In contrast, in a study of 12 healthy nonsmokers (9 men, 3 women) exposed acutely to secondhand smoke (smoke from three cigarettes for 15 minutes with a clear plastic hood over the participant's head; air was mixed with the smoke to maintain a carbon monoxide concentration of 20–40 ppm) no effects on vasodilation were seen (Kato et al., 1999). Carboxyhemoglobin concentrations increased from $0.53 \pm 0.05\%$ at baseline to $0.79 \pm 0.05\%$ after 30 minutes of exposure and plasma nicotine concentrations increased from 0.46 ± 0.12 ng/ml at baseline to 1.38 ± 0.47 ng/ml after exposure. Forearm vascular resistance, either baseline or its response to an endolethium-dependent vasodilator (acetylcholine) or an endothelium-independent vasodilator (sodium nitroprusside), was not changed by exposure to secondhand smoke.

Hausberg and Somers (2008) also saw no changes in forearm blood flow following exposure of 16 healthy nonsmokers beyond the changes seen in response to administration of vehicle. A significant increase was seen in muscle sympathetic nerve activity following the exposure to secondhand smoke, but changes were not seen in blood pressure, except for the response to the cold pressor test, heart rate, and plasma concentrations of epinephrine and norepinephrine.

Data from animal studies demonstrate that some components of secondhand smoke—1,3-butadiene and PAHs that include 7,12-dimethylbenz[*a,b*]anthracene and benz[*a*]pyrene—speed up atherosclerosis development, which results from cell injury and hyperplasia (HHS, 2006). In addition, animal experiments have shown that exposure to secondhand smoke for a few weeks significantly accelerates the atherosclerotic process. Constituents of smoke increase low-density lipoprotein (LDL) cholesterol in the artery lining and bind it to the vessel wall (Roberts et al., 1996).

Platelets interact with subendothelial connective tissue, and damaged endothelial cells also play a role in plaque formation. Secondhand-smoke exposure is associated with the build up of glycoaminoglycan and glycoprotein in animal models, which results in atherogenesis (Latha et al., 1991).

Thrombosis

Platelets (thrombocytes) are cell derivatives that circulate in the blood and play a role in clot formation. When platelets are activated, they become sticky and adhere to each other (coagulate); platelets also can adhere to damaged vascular endothelium. Adherence of platelets increases thrombus formation, disrupts the coronary artery lining, speeds progression of atherosclerotic lesions, and is associated with increased risk of ischemic heart disease (Law and Wald, 2003). The acute cardiovascular effects of cigarette smoke result to a substantial degree from thrombosis-related events (Rahman and Laher, 2007).

In humans, platelet activation has been studied by measuring urinary excretion of thromboxane (TxM), a metabolite of thromboxane A_2, which is released when platelets aggregate in vivo. Smokers have higher concentrations of TxM than nonsmokers (Modesti et al., 1989). One study found that the decline in TxM after smoking cessation was not found when smokers used nicotine patches but was found in those who did not use patches (Saareks et al., 2001). In another study, however, smoking cessation yielded similar decreases in TxM excretion regardless of the use of nicotine patches (Benowitz et al., 1993; Ramachandran et al., 2004). The role of nicotine in that effect, therefore, remains unclear.

Experimental research indicates that secondhand-smoke exposure results in increased platelet activation and aggregation. Researchers assayed platelet sensitivity, an indication of platelet aggregation, in human subjects (smokers and nonsmokers). Platelet sensitivity in nonsmokers increased after subjects sat for 20 min in a room where cigarettes had just been smoked (Burghuber et al., 1986) or in a corridor where others were smoking (Davis et al., 1989). In addition, data on rabbits receiving a high-cholesterol diet (Sun et al., 1994; Zhu et al., 1993) and rats (Zhu et al., 1994) demonstrate that bleeding time, a measure of platelet aggregation, is shortened on exposure to secondhand smoke. Some studies have reported that nicotine in high doses activates platelets in animals (McDonald et al., 1973; Nemr et al., 2003).

Inflammation

Cigarette smoke produces systemic inflammatory effects. Although those biological effects have not been validated as predicting differences in tobacco-related injury or disease risk in randomized clinical trials, they have been predictors of future cardiovascular events in observational epidemiologic studies (Lindahl et al., 2000; Packard et al., 2000). High concentrations of activated oxygen species found in tobacco smoke could potentially damage heart muscle cells and lead to inflammation, which can result in additional organ injury.

Smoking is associated with higher polymorphonuclear (PMN) leukocyte counts, fibrinogen, C-reactive protein (CRP), and other inflammatory markers (HHS, 2004). Some in vitro and animal studies report that nicotine is a chemoattractant, enhances leukocyte adhesion, and increases release of some proinflammatory cytokines (Di Luozzo et al., 2005; Heeschen et al., 2003; Lau et al., 2006). Studies of smokers switching to nicotine medications, however, have found that inflammatory biomarkers decline as in those who quit smoking and do not take nicotine; this suggests that the nicotine in smoke is not responsible for the inflammation (Benowitz and Gourlay, 1997).

Venn and Britton (2007) examined the relationship between secondhand-smoke exposure, measured as plasma cotinine, and biomarkers of heart-disease risk—including CRP, homocysteine, fibrinogen, and white-cell count—in 7,599 never-smokers in the third National Health and Nutrition Examination Survey (NHANES III). Subjects with detectable but low serum cotinine concentrations (0.05–0.215 ng/mL) had significantly higher concentrations of fibrinogen (adjusted mean difference, 8.9 mg/dL; 95% CI, 0.9–17.0) and homocysteine (0.8 μmol/L; 95% CI, 0.4–1.1), but not CRP or white-cell count, than subjects with no detectable cotinine. Similar effects were observed in those with high serum cotinine concentrations (more than 0.215 ng/mL). The increased concentrations of fibrinogen and homocysteine observed in subjects exposed to secondhand smoke were about 30–45% of the concentrations in smokers.

Similarly, Wilkinson et al. (2007) used the NHANES III data to examine the relationship between secondhand-smoke exposure and CRP, focusing on never-smokers ages 6–18 years. An increase in serum cotinine of 0.5 ng/mL was associated with an increase in CRP of 0.96 mg/dL (95% CI, 0.93–1.00).

Clark et al. (2008) used serum cotinine concentrations and the NHANES data (1999–2002) to examine the relationship between secondhand-smoke exposure and markers of inflammation in adult workers. Inflammatory markers analyzed included CRP, fibrinogen, homocysteine, and white cells. Serum cotinine concentrations were categorized as below the detection limit, low (above the detection limit but below 0.2 ng/mL), or high (0.2–15 ng/mL). Workers exposed with low and high levels of cotinine had significantly higher concentrations of homocysteine than unexposed workers. No significant differences were seen in concentrations of CRP, fibrinogen, and white cells.

Flouris et al. (2008) explored the sex-specific secondhand-smoke effects on gonadal and thyroid hormones, inflammatory cytokines, and vascular function. After exposing 28 nonsmoking adults (14 men and 14 women) to a simulated bar-restaurant environment for 1 hour, the study found interleukin-1β and systolic blood pressure significantly increased in men but not women. Gonadal hormones, however, were decreased following secondhand smoke exposure in both men and women.

Hyperlipidemia

Cigarette-smoking is associated with low high-density lipoprotein cholesterol (HDL-C), which is a risk factor for atherogenesis. Smoking is believed to exert effects on lipids, at least in part, by the sympathomimetic effects of nicotine (Woodward et al., 2006). Nicotine increases lipolysis and increases free fatty acid concentrations (Hellerstein et al., 1994). Increased fatty acid turnover is associated with overproduction of very-low-density-lipoprotein (VLDL) cholesterol, increased LD cholesterol, and decreased HDL cholesterol. One study reported that nicotine-patch administration prevented the expected normalization of HDL cholesterol after smoking cessation (Moffatt et al., 2000). Studies of smokeless tobacco users have been used to separate effects of nicotine (similar exposure from cigarette smoking and smokeless tobacco use) from the effects of combustion products (cigarette smoke only). The data on lipid abnormalities comparing smokeless tobacco to nontobacco users is conflicting, making it difficult to ascertain the role of nicotine (Tucker, 1989; Wallenfeldt et al., 2001).

Moffat et al. (2004) assessed the effect of secondhand smoke on blood lipids. Exposure of 12 healthy, male nonsmokers to secondhand smoke (6-hour continuous exposure in a smoking chamber with a volunteer smoker smoking six cigarettes at a rate of one cigarette per hour plus nine other cigarettes burned to attain mean air concentrations of carbon monoxide of 12 ppm, and nicotine of 16 μg/m^3) reduced HDL-C, increased the total cholesterol to HDL-C ratio, and decreased the HDL2-C to HDL3-C ratio by 18%, 14%, and 13% at 8, 16, and 24 hours after exposure. No effects were seen on total cholesterol.

Yuan et al. (2007) developed a smoking system that simulated secondhand-smoke exposure and a mouse model to examine effects related to atherogenesis. They found that exposure to secondhand smoke (6 hours per day consisting of 10 minutes of smoking with a 5 minute break for 5 days per week; particle concentration was maintained at 25 ± 2 mg/m^3) decreased plasma HDL-C in the blood and decreased the ratios of HDL-C to LDL-C, of HDL-C to triglyceride, and of HDL-C to total cholesterol. Those changes lead to lipid accumulation in the aorta and lipid deposition in heart vessels and hepatocytes. Smoke-exposed mice also had increased monocyte chemoattractant protein (MCP) in the circulation and heart tissues, increased macrophages in arterial walls, and decreased adiponectin (adiponectin protects endothelial cells).

Other Effects

Research has examined the relationship between secondhand-smoke exposure and metabolic syndrome, a clinical diagnosis whose characteristics include central obesity, dyslipidemia, hyperglycemia, and hypertension, as well as glucose intolerance and diabetes. Weitzman et al. (2005) used data from 3,211 adolescents (12 to 19 years of age) in NHANES III, 1988–1994) and found that exposure to secondhand smoke, as assessed by self-report or by serum cotinine concentrations, was associated with the metabolic syndrome. Houston et al. (2006) compared secondhand-smoke exposure, ascertained by a questionnaire administered by an interviewer and serum cotinine concentrations, and time to develop glucose intolerance in the Coronary Artery Risk Development in Young Adults (CARDIA) study. Never smoking subjects exposed to secondhand smoke had a greater risk of developing glucose intolerance than those nonsmokers not exposed to secondhand smoke (no detectable serum cotinine).

Metsios et al. (2007) exposed 18 healthy, nonsmoking adults (9 females, 9 males) to secondhand smoke (generated by combustion of a variety of brands of cigarettes adjusted to a carbon monoxide concentration of 23 ± 1 ppm) for 1 hour inside an environmental chamber and examined resting energy expenditure, as an indicator of metabolism, and thyroid hormones, both of which have previously been shown to be affected by smoking. Secondhand-smoke exposure increased resting energy expenditure, and T_3 and fT_4 thyroid hormone concentrations.

EFFECTS OF CONSTITUENTS OF CIGARETTE SMOKE

The constituents of secondhand smoke are discussed in Chapter 2. The following section describes the cardiovascular effects of some of those constituents. These data are from experimental studies in cells or animals or, in some cases, intentional human-dosing studies. Some of the effects in cell systems or animals are seen with exposures above those seen in humans following secondhand-smoke exposure. Also, because of the differences in the experiments and the overlapping end points discussed across the different chemicals, it is not possible to parse out or attribute a specific effect to a specific component of secondhand smoke (Smith and Fischer, 2001a). These pathophysiologic data, however, are important for investigating the potential modes of action of secondhand smoke, as well as contributing to the plausibility that secondhand smoke could have cardiovascular effects. Table 3-1 summarizes the effects of these compounds.

Carbonyls

Vapor-phase carbonyls—mainly acrolein, acetaldehyde, butyraldehyde, formaldehyde, and propionaldehyde—are some of the most reactive and abundant constituents of cigarette smoke and as a group are emitted at a rate of about 1,000 μg/cigarette in mainstream smoke (Dong and Moldoveanu, 2004). Because of their reactivity, carbonyls are more difficult to measure and conduct experiments with and so are not as well characterized as other smoke constituents, but they are likely to have toxic effects, including oxidative stress, as a result of their reactivity. Among the carbonyls, the α,β compounds—such as acrolein, crotonaldehyde, and 3-vinylpyridine—are most reactive and therefore more likely to be cardiotoxic than less reactive carbonyls, such as acetaldehyde, butyraldehyde, and formaldehyde. The concentration of acrolein and other carbonyls in indoor air may exceed outdoor concentrations by a factor of 2–20. Concentrations of 20–300 μg/m^3 have been reported in smoky indoor environments, such as bars, restaurants, automobiles, and trains (Badre et al., 1978).

Because of efficient electron delocalization, acrolein and related α,β-unsaturated carbonyls are highly electrophilic and react avidly with nucleophilic cell constituents, such as glutathione; lysine, histidine, and arginine side chains of proteins; guanosine in nucleic acids; and amino phospholipids (Esterbauer et al., 1991). Their high cardiovascular toxicity has been demonstrated in a variety of in vivo and in vitro systems (Bhatnagar, 2004).

Isolated rat hearts perfused with 10 μM acrolein become arrhythmic and stop contracting within 15 minutes (Sklar et al., 1991). Low doses of such aldehydes as acrolein and formaldehyde have vasopressor effects (Green and Egle, 1983), which suggest a potential mechanism for increased

TABLE 3-1 Known Cardiovascular Toxicity of Cigarette Smoke
Constituents[a]

Compound	Cardiovascular Toxicity	Risk Category[b]
Carbon monoxide	Moderate	Suppression of cardiac function, S-T depression in patients with stable CAD
Nicotine	High	Hemodynamic changes
Acetaldehyde	Low	
Acetic acid	Low	
Nitrogen oxides	Low	
Formaldehyde	Medium	Hypertension, atherosclerosis
Benzene	Moderate	Tachycardia, arrhythmia, arterial hypertension
Acetone	Low	
Catechol	Low	
1,3-butadiene	Moderate	Atherosclerosis
Toluene	Low	
Methanol	Low	
Hydroquinone	Low	
Phenol	Low	
Acrolein	High	Hypertension; atherogenesis, decreased plaque stability, increased thrombosis; suppression of coronary flow and cardiac contractility
Methylethylketone	Low	
Propionaldehyde	Low	
Pyridine	Moderate	
Carbon disulfide	Moderate	Hypertension, ischemic heart disease, thrombosis, hypercholesterolemia, arrhythmias, decreased cardiac output
3-vinylpyridine	Moderate	Atherosclerosis
Cholesterol	Low	
Crotonaldehyde	High	Hypertension, atherogenesis, decrease in plaque stability, increased thrombosis; suppression of coronary flow and cardiac contractility
Butyraldehyde	Moderate	Hypertension

TABLE 3-1 Continued

Compound	Cardiovascular Toxicity	Risk Category[b]
Cadmium	High	Endothelial dysfunction, inflammation, atherosclerosis
Lead	High	Hypertension
Benzo[a]pyrene	Moderate	Ischemic heart disease, atherosclerosis
1,3 butadiene	High	Increased CVD risk and atherogenesis
Particulate matter	High	Arrhythmias, atherosclerosis, ischemic heart disease, hypertension, heart failure, stroke, insulin resistance

NOTE: CAD, coronary artery disease; CVD, cardiovascular disease.

[a] The cardiovascular toxicity of most secondhand-smoke constituents is unknown.

[b] Data are compiled from Bhatnagar, 2006; HHS, 2006; O'Toole et al., 2009; and Smith and Fischer, 2001.

systolic blood pressure. Acrolein can form protein adducts and can oxidize thioreduxins in endothelial cells—effects that promote atherogenesis in vitro. Epidemiologic data indicate that occupational exposure to aldehydes increases the risk of cardiovascular disease. The increased risk of atherosclerotic heart disease in workers in plants that produce formaldehyde (Stewart et al., 1990) and the higher incidence of heart disease in undertakers (Levine et al., 1984), embalmers (Walrath and Fraumeni, 1984), and perfumery workers (Guberan and Raymond, 1985) have been linked to aldehyde exposure.

Mechanistic studies show that exposure to aldehydes decreases cardiac contractility (Luo et al., 2007), increases thrombosis, and leads to dyslipidemia and lipoprotein modification (Bhatnagar, 2004). Those changes could acutely and chronically increase cardiovascular disease risk. Like secondhand smoke, acrolein induces endoplasmic reticulum stress and triggers the unfolded-protein response (Haberzettl et al., 2009). Acute exposure to acrolein activates matrix metalloproteases in advanced plaques of apoE-null mice (O'Toole et al., 2009); this indicates that exposure to acrolein in secondhand smoke could destabilize arterial lesions and trigger coronary events and acute MI. Inhalation exposure to acrolein at concentrations found in secondhand smoke can induce endothelial dysfunction in mice similar to that observed on exposure to secondhand smoke (Conklin et al., 2009); this dysfunction was exaggerated on deletion of glutathione S-transferase P (GST-P), indicating that differences in metabolic disposition of acrolein due to polymorphic variations in the human GST-P gene may be a significant modulator of human cardiovascular disease risk due to secondhand-smoke exposure. Aqueous extracts of cigarette smoke, acrolein and crotonaldehyde, each induce neurogenic inflammation by stimulating the excitatory ion-channel transient receptor potential type A1 (TRPA1) (Andre et al., 2008). Those observations suggest that unsaturated aldehydes may be the main causative agents in the activation of airway sensory neurons, which results in neurogenic inflammation and respiratory hypersensitivity. It remains unclear, however, whether respiratory or inflammatory changes secondary to aldehyde-induced activation of TRPA1 could account for the cardiovascular effects of secondhand smoke.

Other aldehydes generated in secondhand smoke—such as formaldehyde, butyrlaldehyde, and acetaldehyde—are less toxic, but they could increase the toxicity of acrolein and crotonaldehyde. It has been shown that coexposure to acrolein with other aldehydes, such as formaldehyde and acetaldehyde, results in a more pronounced decrease in respiratory rate in male Wistar rats than exposure to acrolein only (Cassee et al., 1996). Moreover, such aldehydes as acrolein and formaldehyde are adsorbed on carbon, and this could further facilitate their pulmonary deposition and systemic delivery. That is supported by the observation that acrolein or formaldehyde delivered adsorbed on carbon or simultaneously with carbon is chemotactic for PMNs (Kilburn and McKenzie, 1978) and that coadministration of acrolein with carbon black, but not either agent alone, has a combined effect on the innate and acquired defenses of the lung (Jakab, 1993). Therefore, aldehydes delivered in cigarette smoke if carried on PM are likely to be more toxic and penetrate more deeply than those present in volatile gases.

Butadiene

Butadiene is a reactive component of the vapor phase of secondhand smoke. It is generated at about 400 μg/cigarette (Cal EPA, 1991). Sampling in indoor bars where there is smoking and measurements of personal exposure in workplaces where there is smoking indicate 1,3-butadiene concentrations of 1–4 μg/m^3 (Brunnemann et al., 1990; Heavner et al., 1996). A smoking ban in an Irish pub has been shown to result in a 95% reduction in 1,3-butadiene concentrations (McNabola et al., 2006). Butadiene has known carcinogenic activity (Jackson et al., 2000), and chronic exposure to 1,3-butadiene has also been linked to an increase in risk of cardiovascular disease. In a case–control cohort study of workers in a styrene-butadiene manufacturing plant in the United States from 1943 to 1982, black workers had a significantly increased standardized mortality ratio (SMR) for cardiovascular disease risk (1.47; 95% CI, 1.17–1.77); the SMR for cardiovascular disease was not increased in white workers (Matanoski and Tao, 2002). The atherogenic potential of butadiene has been documented in experimental animals. The studies showed that exposure at 20 ppm accelerates the speed at which plaque development occurs in cockerels (Penn and Snyder, 1996) although the incidence of plaque development was not significantly different between the exposed and unexposed groups. Acute effects of butadiene on endothelial function or hemodynamics have not been reported, and the cardiovascular disease risk posed by butadiene at concentrations present in secondhand smoke has not been assessed directly.

Metals

Sidestream tobacco smoke contains traces of metals including cadmium, chromium, lead, and nickel (Cal EPA, 2005a). The cardiovascular toxicity of trace metals has not been well studied. However, because of their ability to inhibit the electron transport chain and to increase the generation of reactive oxygen species, they could induce cardiovascular dysfunction even at low exposures. Bernhard et al. (2006) examined serum concentrations of metals in young nonsmokers, passive smokers, and smokers. No significant differences were seen in serum concentrations of aluminum, cobalt, copper, iron, manganese, nickel, lead, or zinc in smokers compared with nonsmokers. However, serum concentrations of cadmium and strontium were significantly higher in smokers compared with nonsmokers.

Cadmium, in particular, has been reported to be highly toxic to cardiovascular tissue. At concentrations found in smokers it dysregulates transcription, exerts stress, and damages the structural integrity of the vascular endothelium (Bernhard et al., 2006). Measurements of antioxidant enzymes indicated that the heart is more vulnerable to dietary cadmium than are the kidneys (Jamall and Roque, 1989). Cadmium compounds stress and may deregulate transcription, damage the vascular endothelium, and have proinflammatory properties. Cadmium has also been linked to high risk of peripheral arterial disease (PAD) in smokers (Navas-Acien et al., 2004). It appears to be an important mediator of smoking-induced PAD in that it has been reported that adjustment for cadmium decreased the strength of association between PAD and smoking (Navas-Acien et al., 2004). That cadmium has been shown to increase atherosclerosis in susceptible animal models (Revis et al., 1981; Subramanyam et al., 1992) suggests that it could also contribute to the chronic atherogenic effects of secondhand smoke.

Exposure to lead at low concentrations has been linked to hypertension. A meta-analysis of more than 30 epidemiologic studies, however, found only a weak association between increased blood pressure and increased blood lead in humans (Nawrot et al., 2002). Chronic exposure of rats to lead in drinking water at low concentrations has been reported to increase blood pressure in rats, and the increase was associated with an increase in the abundance of markers of oxidative stress; hence, lead might increase the production of reactive oxygen species and decrease NO bioavailability (Gonick et al., 1997; Marques et al., 2001; Nowack et al., 1993). A similar weak association has been reported between blood lead and all-causes circulatory and cardiovascular mortality (Lustberg and Silbergeld, 2002). Whether exposure to secondhand smoke results in an increase in blood-lead levels sufficient to induce cardiovascular toxicity has not been established. Also, the cardiovascular toxicity of low concentrations of chromium and nickel has not been reported.

Carbon Disulfide

Chronic occupational exposure to carbon disulfide (CS_2) has been associated with an increased prevalence of high cholesterol concentrations, atherosclerosis, and ischemic heart disease. Several studies of workers in the viscose-rayon industry have reported significant excesses in mortality due to coronary arterial disease and cardiovascular mortality (Balcarova and Halik, 1991; Omae et al., 1998; Partanen et al., 1970). Occupational exposure to CS_2 (between 3 and 65 ppm) has been found to be significantly associated with an increase in LDL cholesterol and with systolic and diastolic blood pressure (Chang et al., 2007; Egeland et al., 1992; Kotseva and De Bacquer, 2000). Exposed workers are at high risk for electrocardiogram (ECG) abnormalities (Kuo et al., 1997). Animals exposed to high concentrations of CS_2 (225 ppm for 6 h for 14 weeks) had increased blood pressure and decreased cardiac output (Morvai et al., 2005). The rapid reversibility of the effect of CS_2 on cardiovascular disease indicates that the effect is directly cardiotoxic or thrombotic (Sweetnam et al., 1987). The reported cardiovascular effects of CS_2, however, seem to appear only after long exposure (5–10 years) at high concentrations. It has been estimated, for example, that it may take a cumulative exposure index of 58–220 year–ppm for viscose-rayon workers to develop hypertension (Chang et al., 2007). Although CS_2 has been detected in secondhand smoke, the concentration measured was several orders of magnitude lower than its permissible exposure limit of 10 ppm. Nevertheless, the effects of low-dose human or animal exposure to CS_2 in tobacco smoke on cardiovascular disease have not been examined.

Benzene

Tobacco smoke contains relatively high concentrations of benzene. Approximately 30 μg/cigarette are in mainstream smoke (Smith and Fischer, 2001b) and 163–353 μg/cigarette are emitted into sidestream smoke. Workers occupationally exposed to high concentrations of benzene have an increased prevalence of arterial hypertension and pathologic ECG changes related to conduction defects and repolarization disturbances (Kotseva and Popov, 1998). Excessive cardiovascular disease risk in commercial press workers (Zoloth et al., 1986) and perfume-industry employees (Guberan and Raymond, 1985) has also been linked to exposure to solvents that include benzene. Subacute poisoning with benzene causes disorders in repolarization and arrhythmia as measured by ECG (Morvai et al., 1976). In rats, benzene increases ventricular tachycardia induced by epinephrine (Juhasz and Bodor, 2000). Benzene also increases the number of ectopic ventricular beats after induction of arrhythmia produced by coronary ligation or aconitine (Magos et al., 1990). Rats and guinea pigs inhaling benzene vapor develop ventricular tachycardia (Tripathi and Thomas, 1986).

The effects of exposure of humans or animals to doses of benzene relevant to those derived from secondhand smoke are unknown.

Nicotine

Nicotine has the potential to have adverse effects on cardiovascular function, although the magnitude of its contribution to cardiovascular disease caused by smoking or exposure to secondhand smoke is uncertain. A contribution of nicotine to cardiovascular events due to secondhand smoke is less likely because the amount of nicotine absorbed in the systemic circulation from secondhand smoke is extremely small. Nonetheless, because we cannot definitively exclude any contribution of nicotine, we briefly review here some of the concerns about nicotine and cardiovascular toxicity.

Studies of users of smokeless tobacco suggest that nicotine is not a major contributor to cardiovascular disease (Arabi, 2006). Users of smokeless tobacco are chronically exposed to as much nicotine as smokers. However, epidemiologic studies have found no increase or small increases in cardiovascular risk in smokeless-tobacco users compared with nonusers of tobacco; in studies that did find some risk, the risk was much lower in smokeless-tobacco users than in cigarette smokers (Arabi, 2006; Hergens et al., 2008; Lee, 2007).

In smokers, nicotine is believed to contribute to abnormalities in lipid profiles. Nicotine, in part by systemic release of catecholamines, increases lipolysis and increases free fatty acid concentrations (Andersson and Arner, 2001; Andersson et al., 1993; Hellerstein et al., 1994; Sztalryd et al., 1996). Increased free fatty acid turnover is associated with the overproduction of cholesterol VLDL, which results in lowering of HDL-C (Therond, 2009). Nicotine is also believed to contribute to insulin resistance via effects of the release of catecholamines (Chelland Campbell et al., 2008); such an effect is unlikely to contribute to insulin resistance in people exposed to secondhand smoke, however, because the nicotine exposure is so low.

Nicotine in amounts delivered in cigarette smoke acts as a sympathomimetic drug in increasing heart rate, blood pressure, and cardiac contractility and in constricting some blood vessels (Benowitz, 2003). Nicotine infusion impairs endothelial function in people (Chalon et al., 2000). Studies in cell systems have reported that nicotine can down-regulate the expression of endothelial nitric oxide synthase, an enzyme involved in the generation of NO, which mediates vasodilation (Zhang et al., 2001). Nicotine also is reported to up-regulate asymmetric dimethylarginine, which would further impair the release of NO (Jiang et al., 2006). Animal studies comparing effects of secondhand-smoke exposure on vascular function found no difference in the extent of impairment of endothelial function between smoke generated from cigarettes with nicotine and without nicotine, and this suggests that the contribution of nicotine was minor at most.

Nicotine might contribute to inflammation by increasing concentrations of intracellular adhesion molecules and vascular cell adhesion molecules, which would result in greater adhesion of leukocytes to blood vessels and thus could promote inflammation and atherogenesis. Nicotine increases secretion of the proinflammatory cytokine interleukin-12 in cultured dendritic cells (Aicher et al., 2003). It is reported to promote release of growth factors, and this could enhance vascular cell proliferation and contribute to atherogenesis (Cucina et al., 2000a,b,c). It has also been reported to promote angiogenesis, which could contribute to progression of atherosclerotic plaques. Nicotine has been shown in experimental systems to release growth factors, including NO, prostacyclin, vascular endothelial growth factor, and fibroblast growth factor (Heeschen et al., 2001; Lane et al., 2005). The relevance of the animal models of effects of nicotine on vascular function to human responses to secondhand smoke is not clear (Hanna, 2006). The effects of nicotine reported in some in vitro and animal studies are opposite the effects of cigarette-smoke exposure. Furthermore, the doses of nicotine administered in many experimental studies are much higher than those seen in smokers and far higher than those exposed to secondhand smoke. Most mechanistic studies involve acute administration of nicotine, whereas tolerance of nicotine develops in chronic exposure, as might be the case with long-term secondhand-smoke exposure (Hanna, 2006). Acute exposures could occur, for example in people who are not routinely exposed to secondhand smoke but periodically visit a smoky bar or restaurant. The contributions of small doses of nicotine seen in secondhand-smoke exposure to human cardiovascular disease, however, are difficult to predict.

Polycyclic Aromatic Hydrocarbons

Several PAHs present in tobacco smoke—including heterocyclines, heterocyclic aromatic amines, and nitro compounds—have been shown to be potent locally acting carcinogens in laboratory animals, but their cardiovascular effects are not well understood. Several epidemiologic and toxicologic studies have provided evidence that occupational exposure to PAHs is a risk factor for ischemic heart disease. In a cohort of male asphalt workers, indexes of exposure to benzo[a]pyrene were positively associated with mortality from ischemic heart disease (Burstyn et al., 2005). The highest relative risk (RR) of fatal ischemic heart disease (1.64) was observed in connection with average benzo[a]pyrene exposures at 273 ng/m^3 or higher. Ramos and Moorthy (2005) reviewed evidence for a role and potential modes-of-action of PAHs in inducing vascular injury and atherosclerosis, presenting data on the formation of PAH-DNA adducts within vessel walls following bioactivation of PAHs. Acute effects of PAHs on thrombosis, endothelial dysfunction, and arrhythmias, however, have not been reported in the literature. The cardiotoxicity of many PAHs and how they might interact with benzo[a]pyrene have not been evaluated, and this adds to the uncertainty in the pathophysiology of PAHs in secondhand smoke.

Particulate Matter

Indoor particles due to secondhand smoke have been categorized as respirable, or "fine" particles that can be inhaled into the lungs and pose health concerns. Sidestream smoke particle size has been reported to range from 0.01 to 1.0 micrometers, with both the mean and median particle diameter in the submicrometer size range (Cal EPA, 2005a). The particles, therefore, are included when sampling is conducted for particles that are less than 2.5 μm in diameter (referred to as $PM_{2.5}$, the so-called fine fraction). In contrast, the particulate phase of mainstream smoke is a concentrated aerosol with more than 5×10^{25} particles per cubic centimeter (Ingebrethsen, 1986), which ranges in particle size from 0.1 to 1 micrometers. Studies consistently indicate that the range, mean, and median diameter of particles in sidestream smoke are smaller than those in mainstream smoke (Cal EPA, 2005a). Secondhand smoke also contains particles that are much smaller (mass median diameter) than the particles in mainstream smoke; however, the characteristics of PM in secondhand smoke change over time due to the "aging process," which includes coagulation, hygroscopic growth, evaporation, condensation, and other reactions (Cal EPA, 2005a).

Many studies cited in Chapter 2 indicate that smoking generates high levels of $PM_{2.5}$ and that tobacco smoke is a significant source of indoor air $PM_{2.5}$ levels in areas with smoking activity. Thus, from those data it can be inferred that typical concentrations encountered where tobacco smoke is present would be up to approximately 100 μg/m^3. Concentrations of 100–300 μg/m^3 should be considered high, and above 300 μg/m^3 would be very high, but observed in some bars and discos. Further data on the effect of smoking bans on indoor air concentrations of PM are presented in Chapter 2.

Mechanistically, a part of the toxicity of secondhand smoke could be viewed as a special case of toxicity that is due to an increase in ambient PM. It has been shown that chronic exposure to environments rich in respirable particles increases noninjury mortality and decreases life expectancy (Bhatnagar, 2006; Brook et al., 2004; Chow et al., 2006).

Time-series data collected from more than 100 million people in 119 cities in the United States and Europe show that for each 10-μg/m^3 increase in PM$_{10}$ there is a 0.3–0.7% increase in cardiovascular mortality (Bhatnagar, 2006). The effects of chronic exposure appear to be larger. On average each 10-μg/m^3 chronic increase in PM$_{2.5}$ has been reported to be associated with an 8–18% increased risk of cardiovascular causes of mortality (ischemic heart disease, dysrhythmia, heart failure, and cardiac arrest) (Pope et al., 2004).

Most (more than 70%) PM-related deaths have cardiopulmonary causes. Specific associations have been reported between exposure to ambient air pollution and ischemic heart disease, congestive heart failure, and arrhythmias. Heart-failure deaths make up 10% of all cardiovascular deaths but account for 30% of cardiovascular deaths related to PM exposure (Bhatnagar, 2006). The Natural Resources Defense Council estimates that 60,000 of the 350,000 cases of sudden cardiac death in the United States each year are related to PM air pollution (Stone and Godleski, 1999). The majority of excessive mortality due to PM exposure attributed to cardiac deaths is similar in scale compared to the risk estimates of exposure associated with secondhand smoke. It has been estimated that exposure to secondhand smoke causes 46,000 (range, 22,700–69,600) excess cardiac deaths in the United States each year (Cal EPA, 2005b). The data highlight the high vulnerability of the cardiovascular system to environmental pollutants and lend indirect support to the notion that both secondhand tobacco smoke and ambient PM contain toxicants with high cardiovascular toxicity.

Further evidence that some of the secondhand-smoke cardiotoxicity is derived from or propagates through a process related to PM comes from several recent studies on PM toxicity. The studies show that PM exposure diminishes heart-rate variability, increases vasoconstriction and thrombosis, induces arrhythmias and endothelial dysfunction, and exacerbates the formation of atherosclerotic lesions in animals and humans (Bhatnagar, 2006; Brook et al., 2004). Similar modes of action have been invoked to explain the cardiovascular toxicity of secondhand smoke (see below). Early work by Aronow (1978) demonstrated that patients exposed to secondhand smoke from 15 cigarettes in 2 hours had elevated venous carboxyhemoglobin, as well as increased resting heart rate, systolic and diastolic blood pressure, and decreased heart rate and systolic blood pressure at angina. A comparison of the exposure profiles of ambient PM and PM from secondhand smoke could also provide some estimate of the magnitude of the increased risk of cardiovascular death, as the committee has done in Chapter 7. One caveat, however, is that because of important differences in composition, secondhand tobacco smoke cannot be viewed as entirely particulate air pollution. It is possible that particles in secondhand smoke are less toxic than ambient PM; however, given that, as discussed in Chapter 2, tobacco smoke contains many reactive components at higher concentrations than in the ambient atmosphere (such as reactive carbonyls, nicotine, and carbon monoxide [CO]), secondhand smoke probably is more toxic and probably has a higher associated risk of cardiovascular death than outdoor $PM_{2.5}$.

Carbon Monoxide

Acute cardiovascular effects of CO in low concentrations are mild, and most data indicate that concentrations present in secondhand smoke do not affect cardiovascular function in healthy young adults (Smith et al., 2000a,b). Early work by Aronow (1978) however demonstrated that patients exposed to secondhand smoke from 15 cigarettes in 2 hours had elevated venous carboxyhemoglobin, as well as increased resting heart rate and systolic and diastolic blood pressure, and decreased heart rate and systolic blood pressure at angina. In addition, children exposed to secondhand smoke have been reported to have increased concentrations of 2,3-diphosphoglycerate (Moskowitz et al., 1990), a compound that is increased in hypoxic red cells; this indicates that exposure to secondhand smoke could decrease oxygen availability and induce tissue hypoxia. In agreement with that view, it has been shown that exposure to secondhand smoke lowered oxygen uptake and increased blood lactate in women engaged in exercise (McMurray et al., 1985). Moreover, atmospheric CO concentration has been shown to be associated with hospital admissions for ischemic heart disease (von Klot et al., 2005) and with increased risk of ST-segment depression during repeated exercise tests performed by patients with stable coronary artery disease exposed to carbon monoxide to result in carboxyhemoglobin levels of 2–3.9% (Allred et al., 1989, 1991). Overall, the data indicate that CO at concentrations present in secondhand smoke is unlikely to initiate atherogenesis or to affect plasma lipoproteins. It also appears unlikely that CO is an important cause of the acute vasoconstriction or increased thrombosis observed in humans and animals exposed to secondhand smoke (Smith and Fischer, 2001b), but it may be important in exacerbating ischemic changes in patients with pre-existing heart disease.

SUMMARY OF POTENTIAL MODES OF ACTION OF ACUTE
CORONARY EVENTS DUE TO SECONDHAND-TOBACCO SMOKE

Exposure to secondhand smoke is likely to precipitate acute coronary events in two general ways. First, long-term exposure to secondhand smoke could predispose an individual for an event by promoting inflammation, oxidant-induced injury to blood vessels, activation of platelets, and possibly adverse effects on lipids, subsequently accelerating coronary artherosclerosis. Supporting the idea that secondhand-smoke exposure accelerates atherogenesis are human studies showing an increase in carotid artery intima–media thickness, an index of systemic atherosclerosis associated with secondhand smoke exposure (Diaz-Roux et al., 1995; Howard et al., 1998). Effects of secondhand smoke on atherogenesis would probably be promoted in the presence of other risk factors, such as family history of coronary heart disease (CHD), hypertension, diabetes, and genetic or diet-induced hyperlipidemia.

Second, in the presence of coronary atherosclerosis and coronary plaque, secondhand smoke is likely to produce acute MI by changing the balance between the demand for myocardial oxygen and nutrients and the demand for myocardial blood supply. Increase in demand for oxygen may be a consequence of sympathetic nervous stimulation seen in response to secondhand-smoke exposure (Hausberg et al., 1997), which could result in an increase in blood pressure and heart rate, as reported in some studies of PM exposure (Brook, 2005; Brook et al., 2003; Delfino et al., 2005), although the study by Hausberg and Somers (2008) did not see changes in those parameters.

An increase in myocardial work usually results in a compensatory increase in coronary blood flow mediated by a release of vasodilators, such as NO, from endothelial cells. Secondhand-smoke exposure reduces the ability to increase coronary blood flow by inducing endothelial dysfunction. That effect has been confirmed in human studies that used coronary angiography to assess coronary artery dilation after administration of acetylcholine and showed artery impairment by secondhand-smoke exposure (Sumieda et al., 1998) and in studies of reduced coronary-flow velocity reserve (Otsuka et al., 2001) after secondhand-smoke exposure. The induction of the chronic inflammatory state on exposure to oxidants in secondhand smoke can result in acute plaque rupture, which can precipitate local thrombosis and acute MI. Sluggish coronary blood flow and a prothrombotic state induced by secondhand smoke may trigger coronary thrombosis with acute MI or sudden death (Figure 3-1).

The pathophysiology of induction of cardiovascular disease by cigarette-smoking is complex and undoubtedly involves multiple chemical agents that are present in tobacco smoke. PM and oxidants such as acrolein are believed to be agents that contribute most to smoking-induced cardio-vascular disease. Results of a number of in vitro studies, animal studies, and human experimental studies suggest that nicotine may contribute to cardiovascular disease by a variety of modes of action but results of human studies involving administration of medicinal nicotine indicate that nicotine is not a major factor.

CONCLUSIONS

- Several components of secondhand smoke, including carbonyls and PM, have been shown to exert significant cardiovascular toxicity. Acute and chronic effects of those chemicals have been identified. The effects appear at concentrations expected to be reached in the secondhand smoke to which people are exposed.
- There is evidence from experimental studies that acute exposure to secondhand smoke induces endothelial dysfunction, increases thrombosis, causes inflammation, and potentially affects plaque stability adversely.
- Indirect evidence obtained from studies of exposure to ambient PM support the notion that exposure to PM in secondhand smoke can trigger acute coronary events or initiate arrhthymogesis in vulnerable myocardium.
- Overall, data on the pathophysiology of secondhand smoke exposure in humans, animals, and cells are consistent with a role as a potential causative trigger for acute coronary events.

REFERENCES

Ahmadzadehfar, H., A. Oguogho, Y. Efthimiou, H. Kritz, and H. Sinzinger. 2006. Passive cigarette smoking increases isoprostane formation. *Life Sciences* 78(8):894-897.

Aicher, A., C. Heeschen, M. Mohaupt, J. P. Cooke, A. M. Zeiher, and S. Dimmeler. 2003. Nicotine strongly activates dendritic cell-mediated adaptive immunity: Potential role for progression of atherosclerotic lesions. *Circulation* 107(4):604-611.

Allred, E. N., E. R. Bleecker, B. R. Chaitman, T. E. Dahms, S. O. Gottlieb, J. D. Hackney, D. Hayes, M. Pagano, R. H. Selvester, S. M. Walden, and et al. 1989. Acute effects of carbon monoxide exposure on individuals with coronary artery disease. *Research Report—Health Effects Institute* (25):1-79.

Allred, E. N., E. R. Bleecker, B. R. Chaitman, T. E. Dahms, S. O. Gottlieb, J. D. Hackney, M. Pagano, R. H. Selvester, S. M. Walden, and J. Warren. 1991. Effects of carbon monoxide on myocardial ischemia. *Environmental Health Perspectives* 91:89-132.

Al-Qaisi, M., R. K. Kharbanda, T. K. Mittal, and A. E. Donald. 2008. Measurement of endothelial function and its clinical utility for cardiovascular risk. *Vascular Health and Risk Management* 4(3):647-652.

Andersson, K., and P. Arner. 2001. Systemic nicotine stimulates human adipose tissue lipolysis through local cholinergic and catecholaminergic receptors. *International Journal of Obesity & Related Metabolic Disorders: Journal of the International Association for the Study of Obesity* 25(8):1225-1232.

Andersson, K., P. Eneroth, and P. Arner. 1993. Changes in circulating lipid and carbohydrate metabolites following systemic nicotine treatment in healthy men. *International Journal of Obesity & Related Metabolic Disorders: Journal of the International Association for the Study of Obesity* 17(12):675-680.

Andre, E., B. Campi, S. Materazzi, M. Trevisani, S. Amadesi, D. Massi, C. Creminon, N. Vaksman, R. Nassini, M. Civelli, P. G. Baraldi, D. P. Poole, N. W. Bunnett, P. Geppetti, and R. Patacchini. 2008. Cigarette smoke-induced neurogenic inflammation is mediated by alpha,beta-unsaturated aldehydes and the TRPA1 receptor in rodents. *Journal of Clinical Investigation* 118(7):2574-2582.

Arabi, Z. 2006. Metabolic and cardiovascular effects of smokeless tobacco. *Journal of the Cardiometabolic Syndrome* 1(5):345-350.

Argacha, J.-F., D. Adamopoulos, M. Gujic, D. Fontaine, N. Amyai, G. Berkenboom, and P. van de Borne. 2008. Acute effects of passive smoking on peripheral vascular function. *Hypertension* 51(6):1506-1511.

Armani, C., L. Landini, Jr., and A. Leone. 2009. Molecular and biochemical changes of the cardiovascular system due to smoking exposure. *Current Pharmaceutical Design* 15(10):1038-1053.

Aronow, W. S. 1978. Effect of passive smoking on angina pectoris. *New England Journal of Medicine* 299(1):21-24.

Badre, R., R. Guillerm, N. Abran, M. Bourdin, and C. Dumas. 1978. [Atmospheric pollution by smoking (author's transl)]. *Annales Pharmaceutiques Françaises* 36(9-10):443-452.

Balcarova, O., and J. Halik. 1991. Ten-year epidemiological study of ischaemic heart disease (IHD) in workers exposed to carbon disulphide. *Science of the Total Environment* 101(1-2):97-99.

Ballinger, S. W., C. Patterson, C. A. Knight-Lozano, D. L. Burow, C. A. Conklin, Z. Hu, J. Reuf, C. Horaist, R. Lebovitz, G. C. Hunter, K. McIntyre, and M. S. Runge. 2002. Mitochondrial integrity and function in atherogenesis. *Circulation* 106(5):544-549.

Benowitz, N. L. 2003. Cigarette smoking and cardiovascular disease: Pathophysiology and implications for treatment. *Progress in Cardiovascular Diseases* 46(1):91-111.

Benowitz, N. L., and S. G. Gourlay. 1997. Cardiovascular toxicity of nicotine: Implications for nicotine replacement therapy. *Journal of the American College of Cardiology* 29(7):1422-1431.

Benowitz, N. L., F. Kuyt, and P. Jacob, 3rd. 1984. Influence of nicotine on cardiovascular and hormonal effects of cigarette smoking. *Clinical Pharmacology & Therapeutics* 36(1):74-81.

Benowitz, N. L., G. A. Fitzgerald, M. Wilson, and Q. Zhang. 1993. Nicotine effects on eicosanoid formation and hemostatic function: Comparison of transdermal nicotine and cigarette smoking. *Journal of the American College of Cardiology* 22(4):1159-1167.

Bernhard, D., A. Rossmann, B. Henderson, M. Kind, A. Seubert, and G. Wick. 2006. Increased serum cadmium and strontium levels in young smokers: Effects on arterial endothelial cell gene transcription. *Arteriosclerosis, Thrombosis & Vascular Biology* 26(4):833-838.

Bhatnagar, A. 2004. Cardiovascular pathophysiology of environmental pollutants. *American Journal of Physiology—Heart & Circulatory Physiology* 286(2):H479-H485.

———. 2006. Environmental cardiology: Studying mechanistic links between pollution and heart disease. *Circulation Research* 99(7):692-705.

Brook, R. D. 2005. You are what you breathe: Evidence linking air pollution and blood pressure. *Current Hypertension Reports* 7(6):427-434.

Brook, R. D., J. R. Brook, and S. Rajagopalan. 2003. Air pollution: The "heart" of the problem. *Current Hypertension Reports* 5(1):32-39.

Brook, R. D., B. Franklin, W. Cascio, Y. Hong, G. Howard, M. Lipsett, R. Luepker, M. Mittleman, J. Samet, S. C. Smith, Jr., and I. Tager. Expert Panel on Population and Prevention Science of the American Heart Association. 2004. Air pollution and cardiovascular disease: A statement for healthcare professionals from the expert panel on population and prevention science of the American Heart Association. *Circulation* 109(21):2655-2671.

Brunnemann, K. D., M. R. Kagan, J. E. Cox, and D. Hoffmann. 1990. Analysis of 1,3-butadiene and other selected gas-phase components in cigarette mainstream and sidestream smoke by gas chromatography-mass selective detection. *Carcinogenesis* 11(10):1863-1868.

Buccelletti, E., E. Gilardi, E. Scaini, L. Galiuto, R. Persiani, A. Biondi, F. Basile, and N. G. Silveri. 2009. Heart rate variability and myocardial infarction: Systematic literature review and metanalysis. *European Review for Medical and Pharmacological Sciences* 13(4):299-307.

Burghuber, O. C., C. Punzengruber, H. Sinzinger, P. Haber, and K. Silberbauer. 1986. Platelet sensitivity to prostacyclin in smokers and non-smokers. *Chest* 90(1):34-38.

Burke, A., and G. A. FitzGerald. 2003. Oxidative stress and smoking-induced vascular injury. *Progress in Cardiovascular Diseases* 46(1):79-90.

Burstyn, I., H. Kromhout, T. Partanen, O. Svane, S. Langard, W. Ahrens, T. Kauppinen, I. Stucker, J. Shaham, D. Heederik, G. Ferro, P. Heikkila, M. Hooiveld, C. Johansen, B. G. Randem, and P. Boffetta. 2005. Polycyclic aromatic hydrocarbons and fatal ischemic heart disease. *Epidemiology* 16(6):744-750.

Cal EPA (California Environmental Protection Agency). 1991. *Proposed identification of 1,3 butadiene as a toxic air contaminant.* Sacramento: California Environmental Protection Agency.

———. 2005a. *Proposed identification of environmental tobacco smoke as a toxic air contaminant. Part A: Exposure assessment.* Sacramento: California Environmental Protection Agency.

———. 2005b. *Proposed identification of environmental tobacco smoke as a toxic air contaminant. Part B: Health effects.* Sacramento: California Environmental Protection Agency.

Caralis, D. G., U. Deligonul, M. J. Kern, and J. D. Cohen. 1992. Smoking is a risk factor for coronary spasm in young women. *Circulation* 85(3):905-909.

Cassee, F. R., J. H. Arts, J. P. Groten, and V. J. Feron. 1996. Sensory irritation to mixtures of formaldehyde, acrolein, and acetaldehyde in rats. *Archives of Toxicology* 70(6):329-337.

Chalon, S., H. Moreno, Jr., N. L. Benowitz, B. B. Hoffman, and T. F. Blaschke. 2000. Nicotine impairs endothelium-dependent dilatation in human veins in vivo. *Clinical Pharmacology & Therapeutics* 67(4):391-397.

Chang, S. J., C. J. Chen, T. S. Shih, T. C. Chou, and F. C. Sung. 2007. Risk for hypertension in workers exposed to carbon disulfide in the viscose rayon industry. *American Journal of Industrial Medicine* 50(1):22-27.

Chelland Campbell, S., R. J. Moffatt, and B. A. Stamford. 2008. Smoking and smoking cessation—the relationship between cardiovascular disease and lipoprotein metabolism: A review. *Atherosclerosis* 201(2):225-235.

Chow, J. C., J. G. Watson, J. L. Mauderly, D. L. Costa, R. E. Wyzga, S. Vedal, G. M. Hidy, S. L. Altshuler, D. Marrack, J. M. Heuss, G. T. Wolff, C. A. Pope, and D. W. Dockery. 2006. Health effects of fine particulate matter air pollution: Lines that connect. *Journal of the Air & Waste Management Association* 56:1368-1380.

Clark, J. D., 3rd, J. D. Wilkinson, W. G. LeBlanc, N. A. Dietz, K. L. Arheart, L. E. Fleming, and D. J. Lee. 2008. Inflammatory markers and secondhand tobacco smoke exposure among U.S. Workers. *American Journal of Industrial Medicine* 51(8):626-632.

Conklin, D. J., P. Haberzettl, R. A. Prough, and A. Bhatnagar. 2009. Glutathione S-transferase P protects against endothelial dysfunction induced by exposure to tobacco smoke. *American Journal of Physiology—Heart & Circulatory Physiology.*

Cucina, A., P. Sapienza, V. Borrelli, V. Corvino, G. Foresi, B. Randone, A. Cavallaro, and L. Santoro-D'Angelo. 2000a. Nicotine reorganizes cytoskeleton of vascular endothelial cell through platelet-derived growth factor BB. *Journal of Surgical Research* 92(2):233-238.

Cucina, A., P. Sapienza, V. Corvino, V. Borrelli, V. Mariani, B. Randone, L. Santoro D'Angelo, and A. Cavallaro. 2000b. Nicotine-induced smooth muscle cell proliferation is mediated through bFGF and TGF-beta 1. *Surgery* 127(3):316-322.

Cucina, A., P. Sapienza, V. Corvino, V. Borrelli, B. Randone, L. Santoro-D'Angelo, and A. Cavallaro. 2000c. Nicotine induces platelet-derived growth factor release and cytoskeletal alteration in aortic smooth muscle cells. *Surgery* 127(1):72-78.

Daisey, J. M. 1999. Tracers for assessing exposure to environmental tobacco smoke: What are they tracing? *Environmental Health Perspectives* 107 Suppl 2:319-327.

Davis, J. W., L. Shelton, I. S. Watanabe, and J. Arnold. 1989. Passive smoking affects endothelium and platelets. *Archives of Internal Medicine* 149(2):386-389.

de Sousa, M. G., J. C. Yugar-Toledo, M. Rubira, S. E. Ferreira-Melo, R. Plentz, D. Barbieri, F. Consolim-Colombo, M. C. Irigoyen, and H. Moreno, Jr. 2005. Ascorbic acid improves impaired venous and arterial endothelium-dependent dilation in smokers. *Acta Pharmacologica Sinica* 26(4):447-452.

Delfino, R. J., C. Sioutas, and S. Malik. 2005. Potential role of ultrafine particles in associations between airborne particle mass and cardiovascular health. *Environmental Health Perspectives* 113(8):934-946.

Di Luozzo, G., S. Pradhan, A. K. Dhadwal, A. Chen, H. Ueno, and B. E. Sumpio. 2005. Nicotine induces mitogen-activated protein kinase dependent vascular smooth muscle cell migration. *Atherosclerosis* 178(2):271-277.

Dietrich, D. F., J. Schwartz, C. Schindler, J.-M. Gaspoz, J.-C. Barthelemy, J.-M. Tschopp, F. Roche, A. von Eckardstein, O. Brandli, P. Leuenberger, D. R. Gold, U. Ackermann-Liebrich, and S. Team. 2007. Effects of passive smoking on heart rate variability, heart rate and blood pressure: An observational study. *International Journal of Epidemiology* 36(4):834-840.

Dong, J. Z., and S. C. Moldoveanu. 2004. Gas chromatography-mass spectrometry of carbonyl compounds in cigarette mainstream smoke after derivatization with 2,4-dinitrophenylhydrazine. *Journal of Chromatography A* 1027(1-2):25-35.

Eaton, M., H. Gursahani, Y. Arieli, K. Pinkerton, and S. Schaefer. 2006. Acute tobacco smoke exposure promotes mitochondrial permeability transition in rat heart. *Journal of Toxicology and Environmental Health—Part A: Current Issues* 69(15):1497-1510.

Egeland, G. M., G. A. Burkhart, T. M. Schnorr, R. W. Hornung, J. M. Fajen, and S. T. Lee. 1992. Effects of exposure to carbon disulphide on low density lipoprotein cholesterol concentration and diastolic blood pressure. *British Journal of Industrial Medicine* 49(4):287-293.

Esterbauer, H., R. J. Schaur, and H. Zollner. 1991. Chemistry and biochemistry of 4-hydroxynonenal, malonaldehyde and related aldehydes. *Free Radical Biology & Medicine* 11(1):81-128.

Flouris, A. D., G. S. Metsios, A. Z. Jamurtas, and Y. Koutedakis. 2008. Sexual dimorphism in the acute effects of secondhand smoke on thyroid hormone secretion, inflammatory markers and vascular function. *American Journal of Physiology—Endocrinology and Metabolism* 294(2).

Giannini, D., A. Leone, D. Di Bisceglie, M. Nuti, G. Strata, F. Buttitta, L. Masserini, and A. Balbarini. 2007. The effects of acute passive smoke exposure on endothelium-dependent brachial artery dilation in healthy individuals. *Angiology* 58(2):211-217.

Gonick, H. C., Y. Ding, S. C. Bondy, Z. Ni, and N. D. Vaziri. 1997. Lead-induced hypertension: Interplay of nitric oxide and reactive oxygen species. *Hypertension* 30(6):1487-1492.

Green, M. A., and J. L. Egle, Jr. 1983. Effects of intravenous acetaldehyde, acrolein, formaldehyde and propionaldehyde on arterial blood pressure following acute guanethidine treatment. *Research Communications in Chemical Pathology & Pharmacology* 40(2):337-340.

Guberan, E., and L. Raymond. 1985. Mortality and cancer incidence in the perfumery and flavour industry of geneva. *British Journal of Industrial Medicine* 42(4):240-245.

Haass, M., and W. Kubler. 1997. Nicotine and sympathetic neurotransmission. *Cardiovascular Drugs and Therapy* 10(6):657-665.

Haberzettl, P., E. Vladykovskaya, S. Srivastava, and A. Bhatnagar. 2009. Role of endoplasmic reticulum stress in acrolein-induced endothelial activation. *Toxicology & Applied Pharmacology* 234(1):14-24.

Hadi, H. A., C. S. Carr, and J. Al Suwaidi. 2005. Endothelial dysfunction: Cardiovascular risk factors, therapy, and outcome. *Vascular Health and Risk Management* 1(3):183-198.

Hanna, S. T. 2006. Nicotine effect on cardiovascular system and ion channels. *Journal of Cardiovascular Pharmacology* 47(3):348-358.

Hatsukami, D. K., N. L. Benowitz, S. I. Rennard, C. Oncken, and S. S. Hecht. 2006. Biomarkers to assess the utility of potential reduced exposure tobacco products. *Nicotine & Tobacco Research* 8(2):169-191.

Hausberg, M., and V. K. Somers. 2008. Environmental smoke exposure: A complex cardiovascular challenge. *Hypertension* 51(6):1468-1469.

Hausberg, M., A. L. Mark, M. D. Winniford, R. E. Brown, and V. K. Somers. 1997. Sympathetic and vascular effects of short-term passive smoke exposure in healthy nonsmokers. *Circulation* 96(1):282-287.

Heavner, D., W. T. Morgan, and M. W. Odgen. 1996. Determination of volatile organic compounds and respirable suspended particulate matter in New Jersey and Pennsylvania homes and workplaces. *Environment International* 22:159-183.

Heeschen, C., J. J. Jang, M. Weis, A. Pathak, S. Kaji, R. S. Hu, P. S. Tsao, F. L. Johnson, and J. P. Cooke. 2001. Nicotine stimulates angiogenesis and promotes tumor growth and atherosclerosis. *Nature Medicine* 7(7):833-839.

Heeschen, C., M. Weis, and J. P. Cooke. 2003. Nicotine promotes arteriogenesis. *Journal of the American College of Cardiology* 41(3):489-496.

Heiss, C., N. Amabile, A. C. Lee, W. M. Real, S. F. Schick, D. Lao, M. L. Wong, S. Jahn, F. S. Angeli, P. Minasi, M. L. Springer, S. K. Hammond, S. A. Glantz, W. Grossman, J. R. Balmes, and Y. Yeghiazarians. 2008. Brief secondhand smoke exposure depresses endothelial progenitor cells activity and endothelial function: Sustained vascular injury and blunted nitric oxide production. *Journal of the American College of Cardiology* 51(18):1760-1771.

Hellerstein, M. K., N. L. Benowitz, R. A. Neese, J. M. Schwartz, R. Hoh, P. Jacob, 3rd, J. Hsieh, and D. Faix. 1994. Effects of cigarette smoking and its cessation on lipid metabolism and energy expenditure in heavy smokers. *Journal of Clinical Investigation* 93(1):265-272.

Hergens, M. P., M. Lambe, G. Pershagen, and W. Ye. 2008. Risk of hypertension amongst Swedish male snuff users: A prospective study. *Journal of Internal Medicine* 264(2):187-194.

HHS (U.S. Department of Health and Human Services). 2001. *Risks associated with smoking cigarettes with low machine-measured yields of tar and nicotine.* Bethesda, MD: National Institutes of Health, National Cancer Institute.

————. 2004. *The health consequences of smoking: A report of the surgeon general.* Atlanta, GA: U.S. Department of Health and Human Services, Centers for Disease Control and Prevention, National Coordinating Center for Health Promotion, National Center for Chronic Disease Prevention and Health Promotion, Office on Smoking and Health.

————. 2006. *The health consequences of involuntary exposure to tobacco smoke: A report of the surgeon general.* Atlanta, GA: U.S. Department of Health and Human Services, Centers for Disease Control and Prevention, National Coordinating Center for Health Promotion, National Center for Chronic Disease Prevention and Health Promotion, Office on Smoking and Health.

Houston, T. K., S. D. Person, M. J. Pletcher, K. Liu, C. Iribarren, and C. I. Kiefe. 2006. Active and passive smoking and development of glucose intolerance among young adults in a prospective cohort: CARDIA study. *BMJ* 332(7549):1064-1069.

Ingebrethsen, B. J. 1986. Aerosol studies of cigarette smoke. *Recent Advances in Tobacco Science* 12: 54-142.

Jackson, M. A., H. F. Stack, J. M. Rice, and M. D. Waters. 2000. A review of the genetic and related effects of 1,3-butadiene in rodents and humans. *Mutation Research* 463(3):181-213.

Jakab, G. J. 1993. The toxicologic interactions resulting from inhalation of carbon black and acrolein on pulmonary antibacterial and antiviral defenses. *Toxicology & Applied Pharmacology* 121(2):167-175.

Jamall, I. S., and H. Roque. 1989. Cadmium-induced alterations in ocular trace elements. Influence of dietary selenium and copper. *Biological Trace Element Research* 23:55-63.

Jiang, D. J., S. J. Jia, J. Yan, Z. Zhou, Q. Yuan, and Y. J. Li. 2006. Involvement of DDAH/ ADMA/NOS pathway in nicotine-induced endothelial dysfunction. *Biochemical & Biophysical Research Communications* 349(2):683-693.

Juhasz, A., and N. Bodor. 2000. Cardiovascular studies on different classes of soft drugs. *Pharmazie* 55(3):228-238.

Kato, M., P. Roberts-Thomson, B. G. Phillips, K. Narkiewicz, W. G. Haynes, C. A. Pesek, and V. K. Somers. 1999. The effects of short-term passive smoke exposure on endothelium-dependent and independent vasodilation. *Journal of Hypertension* 17(10):1395-1401.

Kato, T., T. Inoue, T. Morooka, N. Yoshimoto, and K. Node. 2006. Short-term passive smoking causes endothelial dysfunction via oxidative stress in nonsmokers. *Canadian Journal of Physiology & Pharmacology* 84(5):523-529.

Kilburn, K. H., and W. N. McKenzie. 1978. Leukocyte recruitment to airways by aldehyde-carbon combinations that mimic cigarette smoke. *Laboratory Investigation* 38(2): 134-142.

Knight-Lozano, C. A., C. G. Young, D. L. Burow, Z. Y. Hu, D. Uyeminami, K. E. Pinkerton, H. Ischiropoulos, and S. W. Ballinger. 2002. Cigarette smoke exposure and hypercholesterolemia increase mitochondrial damage in cardiovascular tissues. *Circulation* 105(7):849-854.

Kotseva, K. P., and D. De Bacquer. 2000. Cardiovascular effects of occupational exposure to carbon disulphide. *Occupational Medicine (London)* 50(1):43-47.

Kotseva, K., and T. Popov. 1998. Study of the cardiovascular effects of occupational exposure to organic solvents. *International Archives of Occupational & Environmental Health* 71 Suppl:S87-S91.

Kuo, H. W., J. S. Lai, M. Lin, and E. S. Su. 1997. Effects of exposure to carbon disulfide (CS$_2$) on electrocardiographic features of ischemic heart disease among viscose rayon factory workers. *International Archives of Occupational & Environmental Health* 70(1): 61-66.

Lane, D., E. A. Gray, R. S. Mathur, and S. P. Mathur. 2005. Up-regulation of vascular endothelial growth factor-C by nicotine in cervical cancer cell lines. *American Journal of Reproduction Immunology* 53(3):153-158.

Latha, M. S., P. L. Vijayammal, and P. A. Kurup. 1991. Changes in the glycosaminoglycans and glycoproteins in the tissues in rats exposed to cigarette smoke. *Atherosclerosis* 86(1):49-54.

Lau, P. P., L. Li, A. J. Merched, A. L. Zhang, K. W. Ko, and L. Chan. 2006. Nicotine induces proinflammatory responses in macrophages and the aorta leading to acceleration of atherosclerosis in low-density lipoprotein receptor(-/-) mice. *Arteriosclerosis, Thrombosis & Vascular Biology* 26(1):143-149.

Law, M. R., and N. J. Wald. 2003. Environmental tobacco smoke and ischemic heart disease. *Progress in Cardiovascular Diseases* 46(1):31-38.

Ledford, H. 2008. Drug markers questioned. *Nature* 452(7187):510-511.

Lee, P. N. 2007. Circulatory disease and smokeless tobacco in western populations: A review of the evidence. *International Journal of Epidemiology* 36(4):789-804.

Levine, R. J., D. A. Andjelkovich, and L. K. Shaw. 1984. The mortality of Ontario undertakers and a review of formaldehyde-related mortality studies. *Journal of Occupational Medicine* 26(10):740-746.

Lindahl, B., H. Toss, A. Siegbahn, P. Venge, and L. Wallentin. 2000. Markers of myocardial damage and inflammation in relation to long-term mortality in unstable coronary artery disease. *New England Journal of Medicine* 343(16):1139-1147.

Luo, J., B. G. Hill, Y. Gu, J. Cai, S. Srivastava, A. Bhatnagar, and S. D. Prabhu. 2007. Mechanisms of acrolein-induced myocardial dysfunction: Implications for environmental and endogenous aldehyde exposure. *American Journal of Physiology—Heart & Circulatory Physiology* 293(6):H3673-H3684.

Lustberg, M., and E. Silbergeld. 2002. Blood lead levels and mortality. *Archives of Internal Medicine* 162(21):2443-2449.

Mack, W. J., T. Islam, Z. Lee, R. H. Selzer, and H. N. Hodis. 2003. Environmental tobacco smoke and carotid arterial stiffness. *Preventive Medicine* 37(2):148-154.

Magos, G. A., M. Lorenzana-Jimenez, and H. Vidrio. 1990. Toluene and benzene inhalation influences on ventricular arrhythmias in the rat. *Neurotoxicology & Teratology* 12(2):119-124.

Mahmud, A., and J. Feely. 2004. Effects of passive smoking on blood pressure and aortic pressure waveform in healthy young adults—influence of gender. *British Journal of Clinical Pharmacology* 57(1):37-43.

Marques, M., I. Millas, A. Jimenez, E. Garcia-Colis, J. A. Rodriguez-Feo, S. Velasco, A. Barrientos, S. Casado, and A. Lopez-Farre. 2001. Alteration of the soluble guanylate cyclase system in the vascular wall of lead-induced hypertension in rats. *Journal of the American Science of Nephrology* 12(12):2594-2600.

Matanoski, G. M., and X. Tao. 2002. Case-cohort study of styrene exposure and ischemic heart disease. *Research Report—Health Effects Institute* (108):1-29.

McDonald, T. P., D. Woodard, and M. Cottrell. 1973. Effect of nicotine on clot retraction of rat blood platelets. *Pharmacology* 9(6):357-366.

McMurray, R. G., L. L. Hicks, and D. L. Thompson. 1985. The effects of passive inhalation of cigarette smoke on exercise performance. *European Journal of Applied Physiology & Occupational Physiology* 54(2):196-200.

McNabola, A., B. Broderick, P. Johnston, and L. Gill. 2006. Effects of the smoking ban on benzene and 1,3-butadiene levels in pubs in Dublin. *Journal of Environmental Science and Health, Part A Toxic/Hazardous Substances and Environmental Engineering* 41(5):799-810.

Metsios, G. S., A. D. Flouris, A. Z. Jamurtas, A. E. Carrillo, D. Kouretas, A. E. Germenis, K. Gourgoulianis, T. Kiropoulos, M. N. Tzatzarakis, A. M. Tsatsakis, and Y. Koutedakis. 2007. Brief report: A brief exposure to moderate passive smoke increases metabolism and thyroid hormone secretion. *Journal of Clinical Endocrinology and Metabolism* 92(1):208-211.

Minami, J., T. Ishimitsu, and H. Matsuoka. 1999. Effects of smoking cessation on blood pressure and heart rate variability in habitual smokers. *Hypertension* 33(1 Pt 2):586-590.

Modesti, P. A., R. Abbate, G. F. Gensini, A. Colella, and G. G. Neri Serneri. 1989. Platelet thromboxane A2 receptors in habitual smokers. *Thrombosis Research* 55(2):195-201.

Moffatt, R. J., K. D. Biggerstaff, and B. A. Stamford. 2000. Effects of the transdermal nicotine patch on normalization of HDL-C and its subfractions. *Preventive Medicine* 31(2 Pt 1):148-152.

Moffatt, R. J., S. A. Chelland, D. L. Pecott, and B. A. Stamford. 2004. Acute exposure to environmental tobacco smoke reduces HDL-C and HDL2-C. *Preventive Medicine* 38(5):637-641.

Morrow, J. D., B. Frei, A. W. Longmire, J. M. Gaziano, S. M. Lynch, Y. Shyr, W. E. Strauss, J. A. Oates, and L. J. Roberts, 2nd. 1995. Increase in circulating products of lipid peroxidation (F2-isoprostanes) in smokers. Smoking as a cause of oxidative damage. *New England Journal of Medicine* 332(18):1198-1203.

Morvai, V., A. Hudak, G. Ungvary, and B. Varga. 1976. ECG changes in benzene, toluene and xylene poisoned rats. *Acta Medica Academiae Scientarium Hungaricae* 33(3):275-286.

Morvai, V., E. Szakmary, and G. Ungvary. 2005. The effects of carbon disulfide and ethanol on the circulatory system of rats. *Journal of Toxicology & Environmental Health Part A* 68(10):797-809.

Moskowitz, W. B., M. Mosteller, R. M. Schieken, R. Bossano, J. K. Hewitt, J. N. Bodurtha, and J. P. Segrest. 1990. Lipoprotein and oxygen transport alterations in passive smoking preadolescent children. The MCV Twin Study. *Circulation* 81(2):586-592.

Navas-Acien, A., E. Selvin, A. R. Sharrett, E. Calderon-Aranda, E. Silbergeld, and E. Guallar. 2004. Lead, cadmium, smoking, and increased risk of peripheral arterial disease. *Circulation* 109(25):3196-3201.

Nawrot, T. S., L. Thijs, E. M. Den Hond, H. A. Roels, and J. A. Staessen. 2002. An epidemiological re-appraisal of the association between blood pressure and blood lead: A meta-analysis. *Journal of Human Hypertension* 16(2):123-131.

Nemr, R., B. Lasserre, and R. Chahine. 2003. Effects of nicotine on thromboxane/prostacyclin balance in myocardial ischemia. *Prostaglandins Leukotrienes & Essential Fatty Acids* 68(3):191-195.

Neunteufl, T., U. Priglinger, S. Heher, M. Zehetgruber, G. Soregi, S. Lehr, K. Huber, G. Maurer, F. Weidinger, and K. Kostner. 2000. Effects of vitamin E on chronic and acute endothelial dysfunction in smokers. *Journal of the American College of Cardiology* 35(2):277-283.

Nicod, P., R. Rehr, M. D. Winniford, W. B. Campbell, B. G. Firth, and L. D. Hillis. 1984. Acute systemic and coronary hemodynamic and serologic responses to cigarette smoking in long-term smokers with atherosclerotic coronary artery disease. *Journal of the American College of Cardiology* 4(5):964-971.

Nowack, R., D. Fliser, J. Richter, C. Horne, E. Mutschler, and E. Ritz. 1993. Effects of angiotensin-converting enzyme inhibition on renal sodium handling after furosemide injection. *The Clinical Investigator* 71(8):622-627.

NRC (National Research Council). 1986. *Environmental tobacco smoke: Measuring exposures and assessing health effects*. Washington, DC: National Academy Press.

Omae, K., T. Takebayashi, T. Nomiyama, C. Ishizuka, H. Nakashima, T. Uemura, S. Tanaka, T. Yamauchi, T. O'Uchi, Y. Horichi, and H. Sakurai. 1998. Cross sectional observation of the effects of carbon disulphide on arteriosclerosis in rayon manufacturing workers. *Occupational & Environmental Medicine* 55(7):468-472.

O'Toole, T. E., Y. T. Zheng, J. Hellmann, D. J. Conklin, O. Barski, and A. Bhatnagar. 2009. Acrolein activates matrix metalloproteinases by increasing reactive oxygen species in macrophages. *Toxicology and Applied Pharmacology* 236(2):194-201.

Otsuka, R., H. Watanabe, K. Hirata, K. Tokai, T. Muro, M. Yoshiyama, K. Takeuchi, and J. Yoshikawa. 2001. Acute effects of passive smoking on the coronary circulation in healthy young adults. *JAMA* 286(4):436-441.

Packard, C. J., D. S. O'Reilly, M. J. Caslake, A. D. McMahon, I. Ford, J. Cooney, C. H. Macphee, K. E. Suckling, M. Krishna, F. E. Wilkinson, A. Rumley, and G. D. Lowe. 2000. Lipoprotein-associated phospholipase A2 as an independent predictor of coronary heart disease. West of Scotland coronary prevention study group. *New England Journal of Medicine* 343(16):1148-1155.

Partanen, T., S. Hernberg, C. H. Nordman, and P. Sumari. 1970. Coronary heart disease among workers exposed to carbon disulphide. *British Journal of Industrial Medicine* 27(4):313-325.

Penn, A., and C. A. Snyder. 1996. Butadiene inhalation accelerates arteriosclerotic plaque development in cockerels. *Toxicology* 113(1-3):351-354.

Pilz, H., A. Oguogho, F. Chehne, G. Lupattelli, B. Palumbo, and H. Sinzinger. 2000. Quitting cigarette smoking results in a fast improvement of in vivo oxidation injury (determined via plasma, serum and urinary isoprostane). *Thrombosis Research* 99(3):209-221.

Pope, C. A., 3rd, R. T. Burnett, G. D. Thurston, M. J. Thun, E. E. Calle, D. Krewski, and J. J. Godleski. 2004. Cardiovascular mortality and long-term exposure to particulate air pollution: Epidemiological evidence of general pathophysiological pathways of disease. *Circulation* 109(1):71-77.

Probst-Hensch, N. M., M. Imboden, D. Felber Dietrich, J. C. Barthelemy, U. Ackermann-Liebrich, W. Berger, J. M. Gaspoz, and J. Schwartz. 2008. Glutathione S-transferase polymorphisms, passive smoking, obesity, and heart rate variability in nonsmokers. *Environmental Health Perspectives* 116(11):1494-1499.

Rahman, M. M., and I. Laher. 2007. Structural and functional alteration of blood vessels caused by cigarette smoking: An overview of molecular mechanisms. *Current Vascular Pharmacology* 5(4):276-292.

Raitakari, O. T., M. R. Adams, R. J. McCredie, K. A. Griffiths, R. Stocker, and D. S. Celermajer. 2000. Oral vitamin C and endothelial function in smokers: Short-term improvement, but no sustained beneficial effect. *Journal of the American College of Cardiology* 35(6):1616-1621.

Ramachandran, J., D. Rubenstein, D. Bluestein, and J. Jesty. 2004. Activation of platelets exposed to shear stress in the presence of smoke extracts of low-nicotine and zero-nicotine cigarettes: The protective effect of nicotine. *Nicotine & Tobacco Research* 6(5):835-841.

Ramos, K. S., and B. Moorthy. 2005. Bioactivation of polycyclic aromatic hydrocarbon carcinogens within the vascular wall: Implications for human atherogenesis. *Drug Metabolism Reviews* 37(4):595-610.

Raupach, T., K. Schafer, S. Konstantinides, and S. Andreas. 2006. Secondhand smoke as an acute threat for the cardiovascular system: A change in paradigm. *European Heart Journal* 27(4):386-392.

Revis, N. W., A. R. Zinsmeister, and R. Bull. 1981. Atherosclerosis and hypertension induction by lead and cadmium ions: An effect prevented by calcium ion. *Proceedings of the National Academy of Sciences of the United States of America* 78(10):6494-6498.

Roberts, K. A., A. A. Rezai, K. E. Pinkerton, and J. C. Rutledge. 1996. Effect of environmental tobacco smoke on LDL accumulation in the artery wall. *Circulation* 94(9):2248-2253.

Rocchi, E., F. Bursi, P. Ventura, A. Ronzoni, C. Gozzi, G. Casalgrandi, L. Marri, R. Rossi, and M. G. Modena. 2007. Anti- and pro-oxidant factors and endothelial dysfunction in chronic cigarette smokers with coronary heart disease. *European Journal of Internal Medicine* 18(4):314-320.

Saareks, V., P. Ylitalo, J. Alanko, I. Mucha, and A. Riutta. 2001. Effects of smoking cessation and nicotine substitution on systemic eicosanoid production in man. *Naunyn-Schmiedebergs Archives of Pharmacology* 363(5):556-561.

Sklar, J. L., P. G. Anderson, and P. J. Boor. 1991. Allylamine and acrolein toxicity in perfused rat hearts. *Toxicology & Applied Pharmacology* 107(3):535-544.

Smith, C. J., and T. H. Fischer. 2001. Particulate and vapor phase constituents of cigarette mainstream smoke and risk of myocardial infarction. *Atherosclerosis* 158(2):257-267.

Smith, C. J., T. A. Perfetti, M. A. Mullens, A. Rodgman, and D. J. Doolittle. 2000a. "IARC Group 2B carcinogens" reported in cigarette mainstream smoke. *Food & Chemical Toxicology* 38(9):825-848.

Smith, C. J., T. A. Perfetti, M. A. Rumple, A. Rodgman, and D. J. Doolittle. 2000b. "IARC Group 2A carcinogens" reported in cigarette mainstream smoke. *Food & Chemical Toxicology* 38(4):371-383.

Stefanadis, C., C. Vlachopoulos, E. Tsiamis, L. Diamantopoulos, K. Toutouzas, N. Giatrakos, S. Vaina, D. Tsekoura, and P. Toutouzas. 1998. Unfavorable effects of passive smoking on aortic function in men. *Annals of Internal Medicine* 128(6):426-434.

Stewart, P. A., C. Schairer, and A. Blair. 1990. Comparison of jobs, exposures, and mortality risks for short-term and long-term workers. *Journal of Occupational Medicine* 32(8):703-708.

Stone, P. H., and J. J. Godleski. 1999. First steps toward understanding the pathophysiologic link between air pollution and cardiac mortality. *American Heart Journal* 138(5 Pt 1):804-807.

Subramanyam, G., M. Bhaskar, and S. Govindappa. 1992. The role of cadmium in induction of atherosclerosis in rabbits. *Indian Heart Journal* 44(3):177-180.

Sun, Y. P., B. Q. Zhu, R. E. Sievers, S. A. Glantz, and W. W. Parmley. 1994. Metoprolol does not attenuate atherosclerosis in lipid-fed rabbits exposed to environmental tobacco smoke. *Circulation* 89(5):2260-2265.

Sweetnam, P. M., S. W. Taylor, and P. C. Elwood. 1987. Exposure to carbon disulphide and ischaemic heart disease in a viscose rayon factory. *British Journal of Industrial Medicine* 44(4):220-227.

Sztalryd, C., J. Hamilton, B. A. Horwitz, P. Johnson, and F. B. Kraemer. 1996. Alterations of lipolysis and lipoprotein lipase in chronically nicotine-treated rats. *American Journal of Physiology* 270(2 Pt 1):E215-E223.

Takase, B., H. Etsuda, Y. Matsushima, M. Ayaori, H. Kusano, A. Hamabe, A. Uehata, F. Ohsuzu, M. Ishihara, and A. Kurita. 2004. Effect of chronic oral supplementation with vitamins on the endothelial function in chronic smokers. *Angiology* 55(6):653-660.

Therond, P. 2009. Catabolism of lipoproteins and metabolic syndrome. *Current Opinion in Clinical Nutrition and Metabolic Care* 12(4):366-371.

Thomas, S. R., P. K. Witting, and G. R. Drummond. 2008. Redox control of endothelial function and dysfunction: Molecular mechanisms and therapeutic opportunities. *Antioxidants & Redox Signaling* 10(10):1713-1765.

Tripathi, R. M., and G. P. Thomas. 1986. A simple method for the production of ventricular tachycardia in the rat and guinea pig. *Journal of Pharmacological Methods* 15(3):279-282.

Tucker, L. A. 1989. Use of smokeless tobacco, cigarette smoking, and hypercholesterolemia. *American Journal of Public Health* 79(8):1048-1050.

Venn, A., and J. Britton. 2007. Exposure to secondhand smoke and biomarkers of cardiovascular disease risk in never-smoking adults. *Circulation* 115(8):990-995.

von Klot, S., A. Peters, P. Aalto, T. Bellander, N. Berglind, D. D'Ippoliti, R. Elosua, A. Hormann, M. Kulmala, T. Lanki, H. Lowel, J. Pekkanen, S. Picciotto, J. Sunyer, and F. Forastiere. 2005. Ambient air pollution is associated with increased risk of hospital cardiac readmissions of myocardial infarction survivors in five european cities. *Circulation* 112(20):3073-3079.

Wallenfeldt, K., J. Hulthe, L. Bokemark, J. Wikstrand, and B. Fagerberg. 2001. Carotid and femoral atherosclerosis, cardiovascular risk factors and C-reactive protein in relation to smokeless tobacco use or smoking in 58-year-old men. *Journal of Internal Medicine* 250(6):492-501.

Walrath, J., and J. F. Fraumeni, Jr. 1984. Cancer and other causes of death among embalmers. *Cancer Research* 44(10):4638-4641.

Wang, T. J. 2008. New cardiovascular risk factors exist, but are they clinically useful? *European Heart Journal* 29(4):441-444.

Weitzman, M., S. Cook, P. Auinger, T. A. Florin, S. Daniels, M. Nguyen, and J. P. Winickoff. 2005. Tobacco smoke exposure is associated with the metabolic syndrome in adolescents. *Circulation* 112(6):862-869.

WHO (World Health Organization). 2007. *The scientific basis of tobacco product regulation: Report of a WHO study group.* Geneva, Switzerland: World Health Organization.

Wilkinson, J. D., D. J. Lee, and K. L. Arheart. 2007. Secondhand smoke exposure and C-reactive protein levels in youth. *Nicotine and Tobacco Research* 9(2):305-307.

Winniford, M. D., K. R. Wheelan, M. S. Kremers, V. Ugolini, E. van den Berg, Jr., E. H. Niggemann, D. E. Jansen, and L. D. Hillis. 1986. Smoking-induced coronary vasoconstriction in patients with atherosclerotic coronary artery disease: Evidence for adrenergically mediated alterations in coronary artery tone. *Circulation* 73(4):662-667.

Woodward, M., A. Rumley, C. Rumley, S. Lewington, C. E. Morrison, and G. D. Lowe. 2006. The association between homocysteine and myocardial infarction is independent of age, sex, blood pressure, cholesterol, smoking and markers of inflammation: The Glasgow Myocardial Infarction Study. *Blood Coagulation & Fibrinolysis* 17(1):1-5.

Young, J. M., B. I. Shand, P. M. McGregor, R. S. Scott, and C. M. Frampton. 2006. Comparative effects of enzogenol and vitamin C supplementation versus vitamin C alone on endothelial function and biochemical markers of oxidative stress and inflammation in chronic smokers. *Free Radical Research* 40(1):85-94.

Yuan, H., L. S. Wong, M. Bhattacharya, C. Ma, M. Zafarani, M. Yao, M. Schneider, R. E. Pitas, and M. Martins-Green. 2007. The effects of second-hand smoke on biological processes important in atherogenesis. *BMC Cardiovascular Disorders* 7(1).

Zhang, S., I. Day, and S. Ye. 2001. Nicotine induced changes in gene expression by human coronary artery endothelial cells. *Atherosclerosis* 154(2):277-283.

Zhang, W. Z., K. Venardos, J. Chin-Dusting, and D. M. Kaye. 2006. Adverse effects of cigarette smoke on no bioavailability: Role of arginine metabolism and oxidative stress. *Hypertension* 48(2):278-285.

Zhu, B. Q., Y. P. Sun, R. E. Sievers, W. M. Isenberg, S. A. Glantz, and W. W. Parmley. 1993. Passive smoking increases experimental atherosclerosis in cholesterol-fed rabbits. *Journal of the American College of Cardiology* 21(1):225-232.

Zhu, B. Q., Y. P. Sun, R. E. Sievers, S. A. Glantz, W. W. Parmley, and C. L. Wolfe. 1994. Exposure to environmental tobacco smoke increases myocardial infarct size in rats. *Circulation* 89(3):1282-1290.

Zoloth, S. R., D. M. Michaels, J. R. Villalbi, and M. Lacher. 1986. Patterns of mortality among commercial pressmen. *Journal of the National Cancer Institute* 76(6):1047-1051.

4

Epidemiologic Studies of Secondhand-Smoke Exposure and Cardiovascular Disease

This chapter presents the epidemiologic studies that address following two sets of relationships:

- The association between secondhand-smoke exposure and cardiovascular disease, especially coronary heart disease and not stroke (Question 1, see Box 1-1).
- The association between secondhand-smoke exposure and acute coronary events (Questions 2, 3, and 5, see Box 1-1).

The chapter begins with background information on risk factors for cardiovascular diseases and events. Next is a discussion of the epidemiologic studies of secondhand-smoke exposure and chronic cardiovascular disease. Two other studies conducted following the implementation of smoking bans that address the association between secondhand smoke exposure and acute coronary events are discussed in Chapter 6. This chapter is relevant to Question 1 in the committee's charge (see Box 1-1).

There has been much research on the carcinogenic effects of tobacco smoke and its constituents, but given the typical dose–response relationships for cancer end points and the difference in latency periods between cancer and secondhand-smoke–related cardiovascular effects, the modes of action underlying cancer and cardiovascular effects are likely to be different. In keeping with its charge, the committee focuses on research relevant to the cardiovascular system and does not review the data related to cancer. The 2006 surgeon general's report summarized the literature on the relation of secondhand smoke to the cardiovascular system (HHS, 2006). The committee reviewed that report, and this chapter alone should not be considered a comprehensive review of the published literature. For that, the reader is referred to the surgeon general's report or other recent reports (Cal EPA, 2005; HHS, 2006; IARC, 2004). Recommendations for further research on the matter are presented in Chapter 7.

RISK FACTORS FOR ACUTE CORONARY EVENTS

Clinically manifest cardiovascular disease develops progressively. Extensive analyses of large cohorts show that the major risk factors for heart disease are smoking, diabetes, total cholesterol concentration, and hypertension (Wilson et al., 1998). Additional factors—such as obesity, left ventricular hypertrophy, C-reactive protein (CRP), and family history of heart disease at an early age—have been suggested as contributing to cardiovascular disease risk (Wilson et al., 1998). Data on three large prospective U.S. cohorts followed for 21–30 years indicate that exposure to at least one clinically increased major risk factor underlies 87–100% of cases of fatal coronary heart disease. For nonfatal coronary heart disease, the range was 87–92% (Greenland et al., 2003). An etiologic role of the major risk factors in the development of cardiovascular disease is indicated by extensive studies showing that treating or reducing exposure to risk factors lowers the rate of coronary heart disease events (Chobanian et al., 2003). That smoking is a major independent risk factor for coronary heart disease indicates that its effects cannot be entirely explained by changes in other risk factors and that it increases the incidence, development, and manifestation of cardiovascular disease by pathophysiologic mechanisms that are unique and relatively independent of dyslipidemia, hypertension, sex, or diabetes. Like active smoking, exposure to secondhand smoke could be considered an independent risk factor for cardiovascular disease.

EPIDEMIOLOGY OF CHRONIC EXPOSURE TO SECONDHAND-TOBACCO SMOKE IN RELATION TO CORONARY HEART DISEASE AND ACUTE CORONARY EVENTS

The surgeon general's 2006 report concluded that "the evidence is sufficient to infer a causal relationship between exposure to secondhand smoke and increased risks of coronary heart disease morbidity and mortality among both men and women" and that "pooled relative risks from meta-analyses indicate a 25 to 30 percent increase in the risk of coronary heart disease from exposure to secondhand smoke" (HHS, 2006). This section provides an overview of the relationship between exposure to secondhand smoke and coronary events summarized in that report, not limited to acute coronary events. Much research has been conducted on secondhand-smoke exposure and coronary heart disease and was the precursor to work on the effects of secondhand smoke on acute coronary events. The epidemiologic studies that investigated the relationship are discussed briefly here and then what is known regarding the dose–response relationship and the potential biases and confounding effects that could affect the relationship.

Epidemiologic Evidence

Many prospective cohort studies and case–control studies have examined the association between exposure to secondhand smoke and the risk of coronary heart disease (Butler, 1988; Chen et al., 2004; Ciruzzi et al., 1998; Dobson et al., 1991; Garland et al., 1985; He, 1989; He et al., 1994; Helsing et al., 1988; Hole et al., 1989; Humble et al., 1990; Jackson, 1989; Kawachi et al., 1997; La Vecchia et al., 1993; Layard, 1995; Lee et al., 1986; LeVois and Layard, 1995; McElduff et al., 1998; Muscat and Wynder, 1995; Pitsavos et al., 2002; Rosenlund et al., 2001; Sandler et al., 1989; Steenland et al., 1996; Svendsen et al., 1987; Tunstall-Pedoe et al., 1995; Whincup et al., 2004). They all showed a trend toward increased risk of coronary heart disease associated with secondhand smoke; most but not all of the relative risk (RR) estimates in individual studies were statistically significant. Several published meta-analyses of the epidemiologic studies pooled RR estimates from individual studies and showed a significant 25–30% increase in the risk of coronary heart disease associated with various exposures to secondhand smoke (Barnoya and Glantz, 2005; He et al., 1999; HHS, 2006; Law et al., 1997; Thun et al., 1999; Wells, 1994, 1998). Two recent and comprehensive meta-analyses are particularly worthy of mention (He et al., 1999; HHS, 2006).

He et al. (1999) conducted a meta-analysis of secondhand smoke and the risk of coronary heart disease in nonsmokers. A total of 10 prospective cohort studies and 8 case–control studies were included (Butler, 1988; Ciruzzi et al., 1998; Dobson et al., 1991; Garland et al., 1985; He, 1989; He et al., 1994; Hirayama, 1990; Hole et al., 1989; Humble et al., 1990; Jackson, 1989; Kawachi et al., 1997; La Vecchia et al., 1993; Lee et al., 1986; Muscat and Wynder, 1995; Sandler et al., 1989; Steenland et al., 1996; Svendsen et al., 1987). In all the cohort studies, the outcome was myocardial infarction (MI) or death due to coronary heart disease. Secondhand-smoke exposure at home was measured in all the cohort studies, but only four measured workplace exposure. In four case–control studies, secondhand-smoke exposure was assessed both at home and in the workplace; in the other four, it was assessed only at home. Such incomplete exposure assessment biases results towards the null. Overall, nonsmokers exposed to secondhand smoke had an RR of coronary heart disease of 1.25 (95% confidence interval [CI], 1.17–1.32) compared with nonsmokers not exposed to secondhand smoke. Secondhand smoke was consistently associated with an increased RR of coronary heart disease in cohort studies (RR, 1.21; 95% CI, 1.14–1.30), in case–control studies (RR, 1.51; 95% CI, 1.26–1.81), in men (RR, 1.22; 95% CI, 1.10–1.35), in women (RR, 1.24; 95% CI, 1.15–1.34), and in those exposed to secondhand smoke at home (RR, 1.17; 95% CI, 1.11–1.24) or in the workplace (RR, 1.11; 95% CI, 1.00–1.23). In a separate meta-analysis, Wells reported that the combined RR of coronary heart disease associated with secondhand-smoke exposure at work and not at home was 1.18 (95% CI, 1.04–1.34) in eight epidemiologic studies (Wells, 1998).

The surgeon general's 2006 report (HHS, 2006) updated the meta-analysis of He et al. (1999). The updated meta-analysis included nine cohort studies and seven case–control studies (Butler, 1988; Ciruzzi et al., 1998; Garland et al., 1985; He et al., 1994; Hirayama, 1990; Hole et al., 1989; Humble et al., 1990; Kawachi et al., 1997; La Vecchia et al., 1993; Lee et al., 1986; McElduff et al., 1998; Muscat and Wynder, 1995; Sandler et al., 1989; Steenland et al., 1996; Svendsen et al., 1987). Two of the more recently published studies, by McElduff (1998) and Rosenlund et al. (2001), were identified and included, whereas the articles by Jackson (1989) and Dobson et al. (1991) were excluded because they reported data that were reanalyzed in the paper by McElduff et al. (1998). In addition, the updated meta-analysis did not include one of the two unpublished studies by Butler (1988) or a case–control study published in Chinese (He, 1989). The overall pooled estimate of the RR of coronary heart disease associated with secondhand smoke was 1.27 (95% CI, 1.19–1.36) in the meta-analysis (HHS, 2006). Furthermore, the RR point estimates were similar for men and women and in various exposure venues. The stringent adjustment for potential confounding had little effect on the estimates. The pooled estimate based on the case–control studies was somewhat higher than that based on the cohort studies (HHS, 2006). Most observational studies have adjusted for major coronary heart disease risk factors (He et al., 1999; HHS, 2006).

Five published epidemiologic studies were not included in the updated meta-analysis in the surgeon general's 2006 report (Chen et al., 2004; Panagiotakos et al., 2002; Stranges et al., 2006; Teo et al., 2006; Whincup et al., 2004). Of those, the Scottish MONICA survey is a cross-sectional study (Chen et al., 2004) and so will not be discussed here.

Panagiotakos et al. (2002) investigated the association between secondhand smoke and the risk of developing a first event of acute coronary syndrome (ACS, that is, acute MI or unstable angina) in nonsmokers in the Greek population. A detailed questionnaire regarding exposure to secondhand smoke was completed by 848 patients with a first ACS event and 1,078 coronary heart disease-free matched controls. When age, sex, hypertension, hypercholesterolemia, diabetes mellitus, physical inactivity, family history of premature coronary heart disease, education level, annual income, and depression status were controlled for, nonsmokers who were exposed to secondhand cigarette smoke occasionally (fewer than three times per week) had a 26% higher risk of ACS (odds ratio [OR], 1.26; p < 0.01) than nonsmokers not exposed to secondhand smoke, and nonsmokers who were exposed regularly (three or more times per week) had a 99% higher risk (OR, 1.99; p < 0.001) (Panagiotakos et al., 2002).

Whincup et al. (2004) examined the association between serum concentration of cotinine (a biomarker of exposure to secondhand smoke; see Chapter 2 for further discussion) and risk of coronary heart disease in a prospective epidemiologic study, the British Regional Heart Study. A total of 4,729 men who provided baseline blood samples (for cotinine assay) and a detailed smoking history in 1978–1980 were followed for major coronary heart disease (fatal and nonfatal) over 20 years. The 2,105 men who reported that they did not smoke and who had cotinine concentrations under 14.1 ng/mL were divided equally into four groups on the basis of cotinine concentrations. Compared with the first quartile of cotinine concentration (no more than 0.7 ng/mL), the RRs (and 95% CIs) for coronary heart disease in the second quartile of cotinine concentration (0.8–1.4 ng/mL), the third quartile (1.5–2.7 ng/mL), and the fourth (2.8–14 ng/mL) were 1.45 (1.01–2.08), 1.49 (1.03–2.14), and 1.57 (1.08–2.28), respectively, after adjustment for residential area, age, diabetes, physical activity, alcohol intake, blood pressure, body mass index, total cholesterol, high-density lipoprotein (HDL) cholesterol, triglycerides, white-cell count, forced expiratory volume, and preexisting coronary heart disease (Whincup et al., 2004). RRs for coronary heart disease (for cotinine of 0.8–14 ng/mL versus under 0.6 ng/mL) were particularly increased during the first 5-year followup period (3.73; 1.32–10.58) and the second 5-year followup period (1.95; 1.09–3.48). This study used a biomarker of secondhand-smoke exposure, which is more objective than self-reporting, and found a greater excess risk of coronary heart disease than studies that used self-reported exposure. It is possible, therefore, that the effects of secondhand smoke may have been underestimated in earlier studies that relied on self-reporting.

The INTERHEART study examined the relationship between secondhand smoke exposure and acute MI (Teo et al., 2006). The INTERHEART study is a standardized case–control study of 15,152 cases of first acute MI and 14,820 age- and sex-matched controls. Cases and controls were from 262 centers in 52 countries in Asia, Europe, Middle East Crescent, Africa, Australia, North America, and South America. After exclusions (individuals with unstable angina alone, unconfirmed acute MI, previous acute MI, missing data on tobacco use, or other missing information), there were a total of 12,133 cases and 14,435 controls. Secondhand-smoke exposure was self-reported during interviews with trained staff as times per day, average number of hours per week over the previous 12 months, and smoking habits of spouses; no cotinine measurements were presented. Other factors recorded include: serum apo-lipoprotein B and A1 concentrations, height, weight, waist and hip circumference, blood pressure, heart rate, dietary patterns, physical activity, alcohol consumption, education, income, psychosocial factors, personal and family history of cardiovascular disease, hypertension, and diabetes mellitus. Exposure to secondhand smoke increased the risk of a nonfatal acute MI in a graded manner, with an adjusted odds ratio (OR; adjusted for age, sex, region, physical activity, and consumption of fruits, vegetables, and alcohol) of 1.24 (95% CI, 1.17–1.32) and 1.62 (95% CI, 1.45–1.81) in those least exposed (1–7 h of exposure per week) and most exposed (≥22 h of exposure per week), respectively, compared to never-smokers who were not exposed to secondhand smoke. The overall population attributable risk for never-smokers who were exposed to secondhand smoke for 1 hour per week or longer was 15.4% (95% CI, 12.1–19.3). Those ORs for secondhand smoke compare to an overall OR for current smokers compared to never-smokers of 2.95 (95% CI, 2.77–3.14). The risks increased with the number of cigarettes smoked, from an OR of 1.63 (95% CI, 1.45–1.82) for individuals smoking one to nine cigarettes a day to an OR of 4.59 (95% CI, 4.21–5.00) for individuals smoking 20 or more cigarettes a day. Regression analysis demonstrated a dose response in current smokers with the risk of acute MI increasing by 1.056 (95% CI, 1.05–1.06) for every additional cigarette smoked per day.

Stranges et al. (2006) examined lifetime cumulative exposure to secondhand smoke and risk of acute MI in never-smokers. The authors used data from the Western New York Health Study collected from 1995 to 2001 to examine risk factors for coronary heart disease. Cases were recruited from hospitals in Erie and Niagara counties, New York, after discharge for an acute MI incident (*ICD-9* 410). Controls were randomly selected from residents of those two counties who were ages 35 to 70 years using driver's license lists (65 years of age or under) and Medicaid and Medicare lists (>65). A total of 1,197 cases (64.3% of identified and eligible cases) and 2,850 controls (59.5% of identified and eligible controls) were interviewed. Of those, Stranges et al. (2006) analyzed 284 nonsmoking cases and 1,257 nonsmoking controls, with smoking status determined by self report during interviews. Interviews included medical history and lifestyle habits, and personal lifetime exposure to secondhand smoke in the home, workplace and other public settings. Information was asked according to exposures younger than 21 years of age, and for each decade of adult life (21–30, 31–40, etc.). Information included the number of people living with the participant who smoked (cigarettes, cigars, or pipes) and the number of years the smoker resided with the participant. From that, cumulative exposure at home was calculated by adding the person-years across each age period. Similarly, the number of years working near coworkers who smoked was also calculated. For other public exposures, the number of times per week in a typical month the participant visited bars, restaurants, or other settings in which smokers were present was calculated for each age period. Complete smoke exposure histories were available for 1,478 participants (254 cases and 1,224 controls). ORs were calculated based on tertiles of exposure, both overall and by sex; no range of exposures or cotinine concentrations were presented. Data were not adjusted or analyzed with regard to how recent exposures had occurred. Consistent with other data presented in Chapter 3, data in Stranges et al. (2006) indicate that exposures have decreased over time, especially in the home and workplace. After adjusting for age, sex, education, body mass index, race, alcohol intake, physical activity, hypertension, diabetes mellitus, and hypercholesterolemia, exposure to secondhand smoke was not significantly associated with increased risk for MI, with an OR for those in the highest tertile of exposure relative to those in the lowest tertile of exposure of 1.19 (95% CI, 0.78–1.82). This study does differ from others in that it assessed lifetime cumulative exposures, not recent exposures. To the extent that the effects of secondhand-smoke exposure on CVD are due to recent exposures, cumulative exposure is an inappropriate exposure metric.

Dose–Response Association

A dose–response association between secondhand smoke and the risk of coronary heart disease was reported in several epidemiologic studies and meta-analyses (He et al., 1999; HHS, 2006). In the meta-analysis by He et al. (1999) studies that provided RR estimates of association stratified by the intensity of exposure to secondhand smoke, determined by the number of cigarettes smoked per day by a cohabitant or duration of living with a smoker cohabitant (typically measured in years), were used to generate pooled estimates for the dose–response analysis. The RRs of coronary heart disease increased significantly with exposure to a higher level or a longer duration of secondhand smoke (He et al., 1999). For example, as compared with nonsmokers who were not exposed to smoke, nonsmokers who were exposed to 1 to 19 cigarettes per day and to 20 or more cigarettes per day had RRs of coronary heart disease of 1.23 (95% CI, 1.13–1.34) and 1.31 (95% CI, 1.21–1.42), respectively (p = 0.006 for linear trend). Likewise, as compared with nonsmokers who were not exposed to cigarette smoke, nonsmokers who were exposed to a spouse's smoke for 1 to 9 years, 10 to 19 years, and 20 or more years had RRs of coronary heart disease of 1.18 (95% CI, 0.98–1.42), 1.31 (95% CI, 1.11–1.55), and 1.29 (95% CI, 1.16–1.43), respectively (p = 0.01 for linear trend). A similar dose–response association between secondhand smoke and the risk of coronary heart disease was reported in the 2006 surgeon general's report (HHS, 2006). Compared with unexposed nonsmokers, nonsmokers exposed to levels of secondhand smoke ranging from low to moderate (1 to 14 or 1 to 19 cigarettes per day) had an RR of 1.16 (95% CI, 1.03–1.32). Nonsmokers exposed to levels ranging from moderate to high ($\geq$15 or $\geq$20 cigarettes per day) had an RR of 1.44 (95% CI, 1.13–1.82) compared with unexposed nonsmokers (HHS, 2006). The results from Whincup et al. (2004), presented earlier in this chapter, support a dose response between intensity of secondhand smoke exposure and cardiovascular disease risk. In that study hazard ratios with the simplest adjustment (stratified by town and adjusted for age) were 1.50 (95% CI, 1.06–2.12), 1.56 (95% CI, 1.11–2.2), and 1.61 (95% CI, 1.15–2.27) for the three highest exposure quartiles (serum cotinine concentrations of 0.8–1.4, 1.5–2.7, and 2.8–14 ng/mL, respectively) relative to the lowest exposure quartile (serum cotinine concentration of $\leq$0.7 ng/mL). The hazard ratio for the highest exposure quartile was similar to that seen in light active smokers in that same study (1.65; 95% CI, 1.08–2.54).

It should be noted, however, that in all those cases an increased risk is seen even at the lowest levels of exposure compared to unexposed nonsmokers. As has been seen with active smoking, even smoking fewer than five cigarettes per day is associated with an elevated risk of heart disease, with risks increasing with increased smoking, but at a lower rate compared to the initial increase (Law and Wald, 2003).

Bias and Confounding Effects

Some methodologic issues—including the possibility of misclassification of secondhand-smoke exposure, the potential for uncontrolled confounding effects, and publication bias—have been raised in the literature (Kawachi and Colditz, 1996).

Several potential sources of misclassification of secondhand-smoke exposure have been suggested (Bailar, 1999; Hackshaw et al., 1997; He et al., 1999; Howard and Thun, 1999; Kawachi and Colditz, 1996; Law et al., 1997; Lee and Forey, 1996; Thun et al., 1999; Wells, 1986, 1998). Some self-reported lifetime nonsmokers may have been smokers in the past, and persons more exposed to secondhand smoke may be more likely to have been active smokers in the past (Kawachi and Colditz, 1996; Lee and Forey, 1996; Wells, 1986). However, that potential bias was unlikely to have a substantial effect on studies of secondhand smoke and coronary heart disease because the extent of such misclassification was minor and the RR of coronary heart disease in former smokers was not high (Hackshaw et al., 1997; Howard and Thun, 1999; Kawachi and Colditz, 1996). In addition, recall bias has been suggested because nonsmokers who develop coronary heart disease may have selectively recalled their exposures to secondhand smoke (Bailar, 1999). However, the pooled estimates of RR of coronary heart disease associated with secondhand smoke from the prospective cohort studies were significantly increased and would not be subject to this form of bias (He et al., 1999; HHS, 2006). Furthermore, a failure to correct for background exposure to secondhand smoke in most epidemiologic studies (because truly unexposed populations were essentially unavailable) might bias the associations with disease toward the null (Ong and Glantz, 2000). Although many of these studies use self-report of exposures to secondhand smoke, a number of studies have concluded that self-report can be a valid method to assess exposure to secondhand smoke (Emmons et al., 1994; Tunstall-Pedoe et al., 1995; Willemsen et al., 1997). Measurement errors due to failure to assess total secondhand-smoke exposures from different sources, failure to obtain repeated exposure data over time, or underreporting of exposures of nonsmokers would bias the association between secondhand smoke and coronary heart disease toward the null (Kawachi and Colditz, 1996). Furthermore, the one study that looked at coronary heart disease risk in nonsmokers that used serum cotinine concentrations as a measure of exposure rather than self-reported smoking history had a higher relative risk (hazard ratio, 1.61; 95% CI, 1.15–2.27) than those that used self-reports, suggesting that misclassification of secondhand smoke exposure is not responsible for the increased risk (Whincup et al., 2004).

Several cross-sectional surveys found that nonsmokers who were exposed to secondhand smoke were more likely to report low socioeconomic status and unhealthy lifestyle (low physical activity and poor diet) than nonsmokers who were not exposed to secondhand smoke (Emmons et al., 1995; Koo et al., 1997; Matanoski et al., 1995; Thornton et al., 1994), but the differences between the two groups in cardiovascular risk factors could not explain the observed associations between secondhand smoke and risk of coronary heart disease. For example, the overall RR of coronary heart disease associated with secondhand smoke was 1.26 (95% CI, 1.16–1.38) when the analysis was confined to studies that adjusted for important risk factors for coronary heart disease, such as age, sex, blood pressure, body weight, and serum cholesterol in the meta-analysis by He et al. (1999). Whincup et al. (2004) also conducted analyses with various adjustments. The risk of coronary heart disease was not greatly affected by the adjustments. For example, the hazard ratio in the highest exposure group was 1.61 (95% CI, 1.15–2.27) with the simplest adjustments (stratified by town and adjusted for age), 1.46 (95% CI, 1.02–2.07) with more adjustments (also adjusted for systolic and diastolic blood pressure, total cholesterol and HDL cholesterol, forced expiratory volume in 1 second, height, and preexisting coronary heart disease), and 1.57 (95% CI, 1.08–2.28) with even more adjustments (in addition to all previous adjustments, adjusted for body mass index, triglycerides, white blood cell count, diabetes, physical activity, alcohol intake, and social class).

Another potential bias might be due to the tendency for investigators to submit manuscripts and for editors to accept them on the basis of the statistical significance and direction of the association (positive rather than negative) of study results (publication bias). Overall, there is no evidence to suggest that publication bias attributable to the omission of unpublished data substantially affected the conclusions of the published meta-analyses of the evidence on secondhand smoke and coronary heart disease. For example, unpublished studies were included in the meta-analysis by He et al. (1999). In their meta-analysis, they summarized 18 cohort and case–control studies and performed a rank-correlation analysis of the association between the standard error and the logarithm of RR. If small studies with negative results were less likely to be published, the correlation between the standard error and log RR would be high and would suggest publication bias. The Kendall tau correlation coefficient for the standard error and the standardized log RR was 0.24 (p = 0.16) for all 18 studies and provided little evidence of publication bias. When the study by Garland et al. (1985), which had a relative risk that could be considered an outlier, was excluded from the analysis the Kendall tau correlation coefficient for the standard error and the standardized log RR was further reduced to 0.19 (p = 0.28) (He et al., 1999). We cannot exclude the possibility of publication bias, but there is little reason to believe that it substantially affected the conclusions of the published reviews or meta-analyses of the evidence on coronary heart disease (HHS, 2006).

CONCLUSIONS

- The results of case–control and cohort studies carried out in multiple populations consistently indicate exposure to secondhand smoke poses about a 25–30% increase in risk of coronary heart disease.
- A few epidemiologic studies using serum cotinine concentration, an objective measure of individual exposure to secondhand smoke, indicated that the RR of coronary heart disease associated with secondhand smoke was even greater than those estimates based on self-reported secondhand-smoke exposure.
- The excess risk is unlikely to be explained by misclassification bias, uncontrolled confounding effects, or publication bias.
- Although few studies have addressed coronary heart disease risk posed by exposure to secondhand smoke in the workplace, there is no reason to suppose that the effect of exposure at work differs from the effect of exposure in the home environment.

- A positive dose–response relationship between secondhand-smoke exposure, either self-reported or shown by the presence of biomarkers, supports the conclusion of causality.
- Given those findings, the high prevalence of secondhand smoke in the U.S. general population has important implications for public health.

REFERENCES

Bailar, J. C., 3rd. 1999. Passive smoking, coronary heart disease, and meta-analysis. *New England Journal of Medicine* 340(12):958-959.

Barnoya, J., and S. A. Glantz. 2005. Cardiovascular effects of secondhand smoke: Nearly as large as smoking. *Circulation* 111(20):2684-2698.

Butler, T. L. 1988. The relationship of passive smoking to various health outcomes among Seventh-Day Adventists in California. Doctoral Dissertation. Los Angeles: University of California.

Cal EPA (California Environmental Protection Agency). 2005. *Proposed identification of environmental tobacco smoke as a toxic air contaminant. Part B: Health effects.* Sacramento: California Environmental Protection Agency.

Chen, R., R. Tavendale, and H. Tunstall-Pedoe. 2004. Environmental tobacco smoke and prevalent coronary heart disease among never smokers in the Scottish Monica surveys. *Occupational & Environmental Medicine* 61(9):790-792.

Chobanian, A. V., G. L. Bakris, H. R. Black, W. C. Cushman, L. A. Green, J. L. Izzo, Jr., D. W. Jones, B. J. Materson, S. Oparil, J. T. Wright, Jr., and E. J. Roccella. 2003. The seventh report of the Joint National Committee on Prevention, Detection, Evaluation, and Treatment of High Blood Pressure: The JNC 7 report. *JAMA* 289(19):2560-2572.

Ciruzzi, M., P. Pramparo, O. Esteban, J. Rozlosnik, J. Tartaglione, B. Abecasis, J. César, J. De Rosa, C. Paterno, and H. Schargrodsky. 1998. Case-control study of passive smoking at home and risk of acute myocardial infarction. *Journal of the American College of Cardiology* 31(4):797-803.

Dobson, A. J., H. M. Alexander, R. F. Heller, and D. M. Lloyd. 1991. Passive smoking and the risk of heart attack or coronary death. *Medical Journal of Australia* 154(12):793-797.

Emmons, K. M., D. B. Abrams, R. Marshall, B. H. Marcus, M. Kane, T. E. Novotny, and R. A. Etzel. 1994. An evaluation of the relationship between self-report and biochemical measures of environmental tobacco smoke exposure. *Preventive Medicine* 23(1):35-39.

Emmons, K. M., B. Thompson, Z. Feng, J. R. Hebert, J. Heimendinger, and L. Linnan. 1995. Dietary intake and exposure to environmental tobacco smoke in a worksite population. *European Journal of Clinical Nutrition* 49(5):336-345.

Garland, C., E. Barrett-Connor, L. Suarez, M. H. Criqui, and D. L. Wingard. 1985. Effects of passive smoking on ischemic heart disease mortality of nonsmokers. A prospective study. *American Journal of Epidemiology* 121(5):645-650.

Greenland, P., M. D. Knoll, J. Stamler, J. D. Neaton, A. R. Dyer, D. B. Garside, and P. W. Wilson. 2003. Major risk factors as antecedents of fatal and nonfatal coronary heart disease events. *JAMA* 290(7):891-897.

Hackshaw, A. K., M. R. Law, and N. J. Wald. 1997. The accumulated evidence on lung cancer and environmental tobacco smoke. *BMJ* 315(7114):980-988.

He, J., S. Vupputuri, K. Allen, M. R. Prerost, J. Hughes, and P. K. Whelton. 1999. Passive smoking and the risk of coronary heart disease—a meta-analysis of epidemiologic studies. *New England Journal of Medicine* 340(12):920-926.

He, Y. 1989. [Women's passive smoking and coronary heart disease]. *Zhonghua Yu Fang Yi Xue Za Zhi* 23(1):19-22.

He, Y., T. H. Lam, L. S. Li, R. Y. Du, G. L. Jia, J. Y. Huang, and J. S. Zheng. 1994. Passive smoking at work as a risk factor for coronary heart disease in Chinese women who have never smoked. *BMJ* 308(6925):380-384.

Helsing, K. J., D. P. Sandler, G. W. Comstock, and E. Chee. 1988. Heart disease mortality in nonsmokers living with smokers. *American Journal of Epidemiology* 127(5):915-922.

HHS (U.S. Department of Health and Human Services). 2006. *The health consequences of involuntary exposure to tobacco smoke: A report of the surgeon general.* Atlanta, GA: U.S. Department of Health and Human Services, Centers for Disease Control and Prevention, National Coordinating Center for Health Promotion, National Center for Chronic Disease Prevention and Health Promotion, Office on Smoking and Health.

Hirayama, T. 1990. Passive smoking. *New Zealand Medical Journal* 103(883):54.

Hole, D. J., C. R. Gillis, C. Chopra, and V. M. Hawthorne. 1989. Passive smoking and cardiorespiratory health in a general population in the west of Scotland. *BMJ* 299(6696):423-427.

Howard, G., and M. J. Thun. 1999. Why is environmental tobacco smoke more strongly associated with coronary heart disease than expected? A review of potential biases and experimental data. *Environmental Health Perspectives* 107 Suppl 6:853-858.

Humble, C., J. Croft, A. Gerber, M. Casper, C. G. Hames, and H. A. Tyroler. 1990. Passive smoking and 20-year cardiovascular disease mortality among nonsmoking wives, Evans County, Georgia. *American Journal of Public Health* 80(5):599-601.

IARC (International Agency for Research on Cancer). 2004. *Tobacco smoke and involuntary smoking.* Lyon, France: International Agency for Research on Cancer.

Jackson, R. T. 1989. The Auckland Heart study: A case-control study of coronary heart disease. Doctoral Dissertation. Aukland: University of Aukland.

Kawachi, I., and G. A. Colditz. 1996. Invited commentary: Confounding, measurement error, and publication bias in studies of passive smoking. *American Journal of Epidemiology* 144(10):909-915.

Kawachi, I., G. A. Colditz, F. E. Speizer, J. E. Manson, M. J. Stampfer, W. C. Willett, and C. H. Hennekens. 1997. A prospective study of passive smoking and coronary heart disease. *Circulation* 95(10):2374-2379.

Koo, L. C., G. C. Kabat, R. Rylander, S. Tominaga, I. Kato, and J. H. C. Ho. 1997. Dietary and lifestyle correlates of passive smoking in Hong Kong, Japan, Sweden, and the U.S.A. *Social Science and Medicine* 45(1):159-169.

La Vecchia, C., B. D'Avanzo, M. G. Franzosi, and G. Tognoni. 1993. Passive smoking and the risk of acute myocardial infarction GISSI-EFRIM investigations. *Lancet* 341(8843): 505-506.

Law, M. R., and N. J. Wald. 2003. Environmental tobacco smoke and ischemic heart disease. *Progress in Cardiovascular Diseases* 46(1):31-38.

Law, M. R., J. K. Morris, and N. J. Wald. 1997. Environmental tobacco smoke exposure and ischaemic heart disease: An evaluation of the evidence. *British Medical Journal* 315(7114):973-980.

Layard, M. W. 1995. Ischemic heart disease and spousal smoking in the national mortality followback survey. *Regulatory Toxicology and Pharmacology* 21(1):180-183.

Lee, P. N., and B. A. Forey. 1996. Misclassification of smoking habits as a source of bias in the study of environmental tobacco smoke and lung cancer. *Statistics in Medicine* 15(6):581-605.

Lee, P. N., J. Chamberlain, and M. R. Alderson. 1986. Relationship of passive smoking to risk of lung cancer and other smoking-associated diseases. *British Journal of Cancer* 54(1):97-105.

LeVois, M. E., and M. W. Layard. 1995. Publication bias in the environmental tobacco smoke/ coronary heart disease epidemiologic literature. *Regulatory Toxicology and Pharmacology* 21(1): 184-191.

Matanoski, G., S. Kanchanaraksa, D. Lantry, and Y. Chang. 1995. Characteristics of non-smoking women in NHANES I and NHANES I epidemiologic follow-up study with exposure to spouses who smoke. *American Journal of Epidemiology* 142(2):149-157.

McElduff, P., A. J. Dobson, R. Jackson, R. Beaglehole, R. F. Heller, and R. Lay-Yee. 1998. Coronary events and exposure to environmental tobacco smoke: A case-control study from Australia and New Zealand. *Tobacco Control* 7(1):41-46.

Muscat, J. E., and E. L. Wynder. 1995. Exposure to environmental tobacco smoke and the risk of heart attack. *International Journal of Epidemiology* 24(4):715-719.

Ong, E. K., and S. A. Glantz. 2000. Tobacco industry efforts subverting International Agency for Research on Cancer's second-hand smoke study. *Lancet* 355(9211):1253-1259.

Panagiotakos, D. B., C. Chrysohoou, C. Pitsavos, I. Papaioannou, J. Skoumas, C. Stefanadis, and P. Toutouzas. 2002. The association between secondhand smoke and the risk of developing acute coronary syndromes, among non-smokers, under the presence of several cardiovascular risk factors: The CARDIO2000 case-control study. *BMC Public Health* 2:1-6.

Pitsavos, C., D. B. Panagiotakos, C. Chrysohoou, K. Tzioumis, I. Papaioannou, C. Stefanadis, and P. Toutouzas. 2002. Association between passive cigarette smoking and the risk of developing acute coronary syndromes: The CARDIO2000 study. *Heart & Vessels* 16(4):127-130.

Rosenlund, M., N. Berglind, A. Gustavsson, C. Reuterwall, J. Hallqvist, F. Nyberg, G. Pershagen, and S. S. Group. 2001. Environmental tobacco smoke and myocardial infarction among never-smokers in the Stockholm Heart Epidemiology Program (SHEEP). *Epidemiology* 12(5):558-564.

Sandler, D. P., G. W. Comstock, K. J. Helsing, and D. L. Shore. 1989. Deaths from all causes in non-smokers who lived with smokers. *American Journal of Public Health* 79(2):163-167.

Steenland, K., M. Thun, C. Lally, and C. Heath, Jr. 1996. Environmental tobacco smoke and coronary heart disease in the American Cancer Society CPS-II cohort. *Circulation* 94(4):622-628.

Stranges, S., M. R. Bonner, F. Fucci, K. M. Cummings, J. L. Freudenheim, J. M. Dorn, P. Muti, G. A. Giovino, A. Hyland, and M. Trevisan. 2006. Lifetime cumulative exposure to secondhand smoke and risk of myocardial infarction in never smokers: Results from the Western New York Health study, 1995-2001. *Archives of Internal Medicine* 166(18):1961-1967.

Svendsen, K. H., L. H. Kuller, M. J. Martin, and J. K. Ockene. 1987. Effects of passive smoking in the Multiple Risk Factor Intervention trial. *American Journal of Epidemiology* 126(5):783-795.

Teo, K. K., S. Ounpuu, S. Hawken, M. R. Pandey, V. Valentin, D. Hunt, R. Diaz, W. Rashed, R. Freeman, L. Jiang, X. Zhang, and S. Yusuf. 2006. Tobacco use and risk of myocardial infarction in 52 countries in the INTERHEART study: A case-control study. *Lancet* 368(9536):647-658.

Thornton, A., P. Lee, and J. Fry. 1994. Differences between smokers, ex-smokers, passive smokers and non-smokers. *Journal of Clinical Epidemiology* 47(10):1143-1162.

Thun, M., J. Henley, and L. Apicella. 1999. Epidemiologic studies of fatal and nonfatal cardiovascular disease and ETS exposure from spousal smoking. *Environmental Health Perspectives* 107 Suppl 6:841-846.

Tunstall-Pedoe, H., C. A. Brown, M. Woodward, and R. Tavendale. 1995. Passive smoking by self report and serum cotinine and the prevalence of respiratory and coronary heart disease in the Scottish Heart Health study. *Journal of Epidemiology and Community Health* 49(2):139-143.

Wells, A. J. 1986. Misclassification as a factor in passive smoking risk. *Lancet* 2(8507):638.

———. 1994. Passive smoking as a cause of heart disease. *Journal of the American College of Cardiology* 24(2):546-554.

———. 1998. Heart disease from passive smoking in the workplace. *Journal of the American College of Cardiology* 31(1):1-9.

Whincup, P. H., J. A. Gilg, J. R. Emberson, M. J. Jarvis, C. Feyerabend, A. Bryant, M. Walker, and D. G. Cook. 2004. Passive smoking and risk of coronary heart disease and stroke: Prospective study with cotinine measurement. *BMJ* 329(7459):200-205.

Willemsen, M. C., J. Brug, D. R. Uges, and M. L. Vos de Wael. 1997. Validity and reliability of self-reported exposure to environmental tobacco smoke in work offices. *Journal of Occupational & Environmental Medicine* 39(11):1111-1114.

Wilson, P. W., R. B. D'Agostino, D. Levy, A. M. Belanger, H. Silbershatz, and W. B. Kannel. 1998. Prediction of coronary heart disease using risk factor categories. *Circulation* 97(18):1837-1847.

5

The Background of Smoking Bans

This chapter provides background information on smoking bans, including a brief discussion of the history of tobacco policies that led to bans and the current status of bans in the United States and globally. More comprehensive reviews of the history of smoking bans and the scientific evidence and societal forces for and against them can be found in *The Health Consequences of Involuntary Exposure to Tobacco Smoke: A Report of the Surgeon General* (HHS, 2006) and the Institute of Medicine (IOM) report *Ending the Tobacco Problem: A Blueprint for the Nation* (IOM, 2007). The committee here discusses some of the issues around smoking bans that are relevant to the evaluation and interpretation of the literature on the effect of bans on the incidence of acute coronary events. Specifically, it discusses different types of smoking bans; the enforcement of bans; activities which often accompany bans, such as educational and outreach programs; and the effect of bans on individual behaviors, such as smoking.

HISTORY OF U.S. SMOKING POLICIES

The first surgeon general's report on the adverse health effects of smoking was published in 1964 (HHS, 1964). Within a year of that report, the first law requiring the labeling of cigarette packages with health warnings was passed (the Cigarette Labeling and Advertising Act of 1965); it was followed a few years later by bans on cigarette advertising on television and radio (the 1969 Public Health Cigarette Smoking Act). By 1972, another report of the surgeon general, *The Health Consequences of Smoking*, discussed the potential adverse effects of secondhand-tobacco smoke in people with preexisting disease (HHS, 1972). Table 5-1 lists some of the scientific reports and the clean-air policies implemented in the United States since the 1972 report; these milestones are detailed further in the surgeon general's 2006 report (HHS, 2006). Restrictions on smoking in public places, government buildings, and airplanes were implemented in the 1970s, most of which limited but did not ban smoking. In 1973, Arizona became the first state to have some smoke-free public places, and the Civil Aeronautics Board requested no-smoking sections on all commercial airline flights (Koop, 1986). In the 1980s, several reports—*The Health Conse-quences of Involuntary Smoking: A Report of the Surgeon General* (HHS,

TABLE 5-1 Summary of Milestones in Decreasing Indoor Tobacco Smoke in the United States[a]

Year	Event
1971	The surgeon general proposes a federal smoking ban in public places.
1972	The first report of the surgeon general to identify secondhand smoke as posing a health risk is released.
1973	Arizona becomes the first state to restrict smoking in several public places. The Civil Aeronautics Board requires no-smoking sections on all commercial airline flights.
1974	Connecticut passes the first state law to apply smoking restrictions in restaurants.
1975	Minnesota passes a statewide law restricting smoking in public places.
1977	Berkeley, California, becomes the first community to limit smoking in restaurants and other public places.
1983	San Francisco passes a law to place private workplaces under smoking restrictions.
1986	A report of the surgeon general focuses entirely on the health consequences of involuntary smoking, proclaiming secondhand smoke a cause of lung cancer in healthy nonsmokers. The National Research Council issues a report on the health consequences of involuntary smoking. Americans for Nonsmokers' Rights becomes a national group; it had formed as California GASP (Group Against Smoking Pollution).
1987	The U.S. Department of Health and Human Services establishes a smoke-free environment in all its buildings, affecting 120,000 employees nationwide. Minnesota passes a law requiring all hospitals in the state to prohibit smoking by 1990. A Gallup poll finds, for the first time, that a majority (55%) of U.S. adults favor a complete ban on smoking in all public places.
1988	A congressionally mandated smoking ban takes effect on all domestic airline flights of 2 h or less. New York City's ordinance for clean indoor air takes effect; the ordinance bans or severely limits smoking in various public places and affects 7 million people. California implements a statewide ban on smoking aboard all commercial intrastate airplanes, trains, and buses.

TABLE 5-1 Continued

Year	Event
1990	A congressionally mandated smoking ban takes effect on all domestic airline flights of 6 h or less. The U.S. Environmental Protection Agency (EPA) issues a draft risk assessment of secondhand smoke.
1991	The National Institute for Occupational Safety and Health issues a bulletin recommending that secondhand smoke be reduced to the lowest feasible concentration in the workplace.
1992	Hospitals applying to the Joint Commission on Accreditation of Healthcare Organizations for accreditation are required to develop a policy prohibiting smoking by patients, visitors, employees, volunteers, and medical staff. EPA releases its report classifying secondhand smoke as a group A carcinogen (known to be harmful to humans), placing secondhand smoke in the same category as asbestos, benzene, and radon.
1993	Los Angeles passes a ban on smoking in all restaurants. The U.S. Postal Service eliminates smoking in all facilities. Congress enacts a smoke-free policy for Special Supplemental Food Program for Women, Infants, and Children (WIC) clinics. A working group of 16 state attorneys general releases recommendations for establishing smoke-free policies in fast-food restaurants. Vermont bans smoking in all public buildings and in many private buildings open to the public.
1994	The U.S. Department of Defense prohibits smoking in all indoor military facilities. The Occupational Safety and Health Administration proposes a rule that would ban smoking in most U.S. workplaces. San Francisco passes a ban on smoking in all restaurants and workplaces. The Pro-Children Act requires persons who provide federally funded children's services to prohibit smoking in their facilities. Utah enacts a law restricting smoking in most workplaces.
1995	New York City passes a comprehensive ordinance effectively banning smoking in most workplaces. Maryland enacts a smoke-free policy for all workplaces except hotels, bars, some restaurants, and private clubs. California passes comprehensive legislation that prohibits smoking in most enclosed workplaces. Vermont's smoking ban is extended to include restaurants, bars, hotels, and motels except establishments holding a cabaret license.
1996	The U.S. Department of Transportation reports that about 80% of nonstop scheduled U.S. airline flights between the United States and foreign points will be smoke-free by June 1, 1996.
1997	President Clinton signs an executive order establishing a smoke-free environment for federal employees and all members of the public visiting federally owned facilities. The California EPA issues a report determining that secondhand smoke is a toxic air contaminant. Settlement is reached in the class-action lawsuit brought by flight attendants exposed to secondhand smoke.
1998	The U.S. Senate ends smoking in the Senate's public spaces. California law takes effect banning smoking in bars that do not have a separately ventilated smoking area. The Minnesota tobacco-document depository is created as a result of a tobacco-industry settlement with Minnesota and BlueCross BlueShield of Minnesota. U.S. tobacco companies are required to maintain a public depository to house more than 32 million pages of previously secret internal tobacco-industry documents.

Continued

TABLE 5-1 Continued

Year	Event
2000	The New Jersey Supreme Court strikes down a local clean-indoor-air ordinance adopted by the city of Princeton on the grounds that state law preempts local smoking restrictions. A congressionally mandated smoking ban takes effect on all international flights departing from or arriving in the United States.
2002	New York City holds its first hearing on an indoor smoking ban that would include all bars and restaurants. The amended Clean Indoor Air Act enacted by the state of New York (Public Health Law, Article 13-E), which took effect July 24, 2003, prohibits smoking in virtually all workplaces, including restaurants and bars. The Michigan Supreme Court refuses to hear an appeal of lower-court rulings striking down a local clean-indoor-air ordinance enacted by the city of Marquette on the grounds that state law preempts local communities from adopting smoking restrictions in restaurants and bars that are more stringent than the state standard. Delaware enacts a comprehensive smoke-free law and repeals a preemption provision precluding communities from adopting local smoking restrictions that are more stringent than state law. Florida voters approve a ballot measure that amends the state constitution to require most workplaces and public places—with some exceptions, such as bars—to be smoke-free.
2003	Dozens of U.S. airports—including airline clubs, passenger terminals, and nonpublic work areas—are designated as smoke-free. Connecticut and New York enact comprehensive smoke-free laws. Maine enacts a law requiring bars, pool halls, and bingo venues to be smoke-free. State supreme courts in Iowa and New Hampshire strike down local smoke-free ordinances, ruling that they are preempted by state law.
2004	Massachusetts and Rhode Island enact comprehensive smoke-free laws. The International Agency for Research on Cancer issues a new monograph identifying secondhand smoke as "carcinogenic to humans."
2005	North Dakota, Vermont, Montana, and Washington enact 100% smoke-free workplace and/or restaurant and/or bar regulations.
2006	New Jersey, Colorado, Hawaii, Ohio, and Nevada enact 100% smoke-free workplace and/or restaurant and/or bar regulations.
2007	Louisiana, Arizona, New Mexico, New Hampshire, and Minnesota enact 100% smoke-free workplace and/or restaurant and/or bar regulations.
2008	Illinois, Maryland, Iowa, and Pennsylvania enact 100% smoke-free workplace and/or restaurant and/or bars regulations.
As of Jan. 4, 2009	Oregon enacts 100% smoke-free workplace and restaurant regulations, and bar restrictions. Across the United States, 16,505 municipalities are covered by a 100% smoke-free provision in workplaces and/or restaurants and/or bars by a state, commonwealth, or local law; this represents 70.2% of the U.S. population. The District of Columbia and 37 states have local laws in effect that require 100% smoke-free workplaces and/or restaurants and/or bars.

[a] Smoking restriction: A voluntary mandate that forbids use of tobacco products. Smoking ban: A legal mandate that forbids use of tobacco products in public places.
SOURCE: ANRF, 2009.

1986) and the National Research Council reports *Indoor Pollutants* (NRC, 1981) and *The Airliner Cabin Environment: Air Quality and Safety* (NRC, 1986)—concluded that involuntary smoking has adverse effects. Increasing activity of nonsmokers' rights organizations and shifts in public opinion led to implementation of more comprehensive bans, including bans on smoking on some domestic flights and in some government buildings (HHS, 2006). By 1986, 41 states and the District of Columbia had statutes that restricted smoking to some extent, but that were not as strong or extensive as most bans currently in place (Bayer and Colgrove, 2002; IOM, 2007). In 1992, the U.S. Environmental Protection Agency (EPA) released *The Respiratory Health Effects of Passive Smoking: Lung Cancer and Other Disorders* (EPA, 1992), which concluded that "environmental tobacco smoke (ETS) in the United States presents a serious and substantial public health impact." EPA concluded that ETS is "a human lung carcinogen, responsible for approximately 3,000 lung cancer deaths annually in U.S. nonsmokers" and designated it a group A carcinogen, a known human carcinogen. EPA also cited other respiratory health effects in that report. As can be seen in Table 5-1, following the release of that report and with an increasing body of evidence demonstrating the adverse health effects of secondhand smoke, during the 1990s state and local governments across the country enacted an increasing number of more restrictive bans, including bans on smoking in most workplaces in some states. In the late 1990s and early 2000s, some states implemented comprehensive smoking bans that prohibited smoking in most workplaces and all public places, including previously exempted bars and restaurants (HHS, 2006). The first report about the association between cardiovascular risk and secondhand smoke appeared in 1985 (Garland et al., 1985).

According to the American Nonsmokers' Rights Foundation's U.S. Tobacco Control Laws Database©,[1] as of January 4, 2009, "a total of 30 states, along with Puerto Rico and the District of Columbia, have laws in effect that require 100% smokefree workplaces and/or restaurants and/ or bars." It estimated that 70.2% of the U.S. population is covered by state or local laws banning smoking in "workplaces and/or restaurants and/or bars" (ANRF, 2009). Despite those increases in smoking bans, as recently as 1999–2004, the National Health and Nutrition Examination Survey (NHANES) estimated, on the basis of detectable serum cotinine, that 46.4% of U.S. nonsmokers ages 4 years and older were exposed to

---

[1] The American Nonsmokers' Rights Foundation has tracked, collected, and analyzed tobacco-control ordinances, bylaws, and board of health regulations since the early 1980s. The information has formed the basis of the U.S. Tobacco Control Laws Database©, a national collection of local legislation that contains provisions covering at least one of the following: clean-indoor-air regulations; restrictions on youth access to tobacco, tobacco advertising and promotion; tobacco excise taxes; and conditional use permits.

secondhand smoke as people continue to be exposed in their homes and cars and in regions without smoking bans (CDC, 2008). That was a sharp decrease from the 1988–1994 NHANES data, in which the estimate was 84%, and supported an overall downward trend in secondhand-smoke exposure in the United States.

GLOBAL TOBACCO POLICIES

In addition to the United States, many countries (or portions of countries) around the world have implemented smoking restrictions and bans. They include Canada, Italy, and Scotland, where some of the key surveillance studies reviewed by this committee were conducted.

The growing global support for reducing tobacco use and secondhand-smoke exposure is evident from the *World Health Organization Framework Convention on Tobacco Control* (WHO, 2005). First proposed by the World Health Organization (WHO) in 1999, the treaty was adopted by the World Health Assembly in 2003. It commits ratifying nations to "protect present and future generations from the devastating health, social, environmental and economic consequences of tobacco consumption and exposure to tobacco smoke by providing a framework for tobacco control measures to be implemented by the Parties at the national, regional and international levels in order to reduce continually and substantially the prevalence of tobacco use and exposure to tobacco smoke" (WHO, 2005). Article 8 of the treaty commits parties "to protect all persons from exposure to tobacco smoke." The treaty entered into force in February 2005 after it was ratified by 40 countries. As of July 30, 2009, 168 of the 192 WHO member states are signatories, and 166 WHO member states had ratified the treaty and become parties, covering 86.24% of the world population (WHO, 2009). The 2007 WHO report *Protection from Exposure to Second-hand Tobacco Smoke* (WHO, 2007) recommends that member states enact, implement, and enforce laws requiring workplaces and public places to be 100% smoke-free and pursue educational programs and activities to reduce secondhand-smoke exposure in homes.

The data in Figure 5-1, from the *WHO Report on the Global Tobacco Epidemic, 2008—The MPOWER Package*, however, show that "only 5% of the world's population is covered by comprehensive smoke-free laws" as defined by WHO (2008), so much work remains. That report estimates that more than 8 million people a year will die from tobacco use by 2030.

ISSUES SURROUNDING SMOKING BANS

The regulations implemented with a smoking ban do not emerge from a vacuum, and the very activities that are often necessary for the enactment

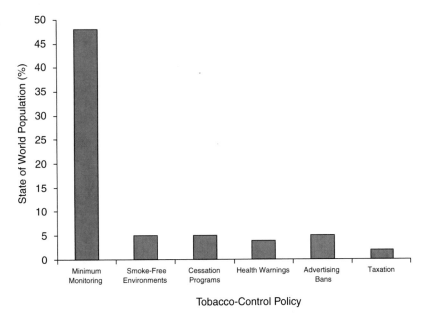

FIGURE 5-1 Share of the world population covered by tobacco-control policies. SOURCE: Modified from WHO, 2008.

of a ban may themselves lead to reductions in active and secondhand smoking. As can be seen in Figure 5-2 (IARC, 2008), the health of nonsmokers after the implementation of a smoke-free policy can be affected not only by reduced secondhand-smoke exposure but also by concurrent changes (such as home smoking bans and decreases in smoking by people in other environments) attributable to increased awareness in the community, increased spontaneous cessation, and higher cessation success rates. The latter factors might have additional implications for the period over which followup is performed because their own timing might influence the effectiveness of a ban. Therefore, in evaluating and interpreting studies of the effects of smoking bans on health outcomes, the other concurrent activities must also be taken into consideration. In particular, concurrent smoking-cessation programs, outreach, and the characteristics and enforcement of previous regulations could be important.

Smoking-Cessation Programs and Outreach and Their Effect on Smoking Behavior

Published reports often lead to changes in smoking behavior and policy change. For example, as can be seen in Figure 5-3, the overall increase in

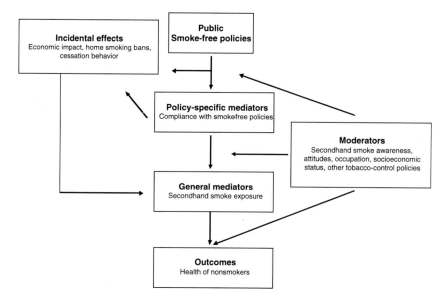

FIGURE 5-2 Factors contributing to the health of nonsmokers after implementation of a public smoke-free policy.
SOURCE: Modified from IARC, 2008.

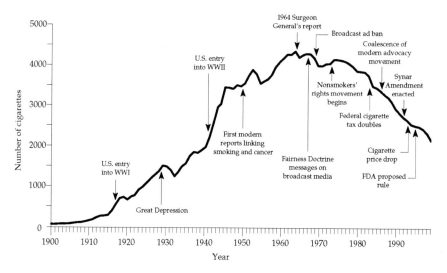

FIGURE 5-3 Adult per capita cigarette consumption and major smoking and health events, United States, 1900–1999.
NOTE: FDA, U.S. Food and Drug Administration.
SOURCE: HHS, 2000.

per capita cigarette consumption in the U.S. population ended after the publication of the surgeon general's 1964 report on the health effects of smoking (HHS, 2000). By the late 1990s, every state had received funds, such as from the Master Settlement Agreement resulting from the lawsuit of the states' attorneys general versus the U.S. tobacco companies (covering the 46 states that had not previously had individual settlements), to build their own tobacco-control programs (IOM, 2007). State and local efforts to implement smoking bans sometimes have a multiprong approach, accompanying smoking bans with media outreach, school-based programs, changes in tobacco pricing, or support for cessation programs.

A portion of the overall decline in smoking prevalence and intensity over the past 25 years can be attributed to general tobacco-control interventions (price increases and stronger antismoking culture). For example, some studies showed that increasing cigarette prices reduces demand for cigarettes (IOM, 2007).

The *WHO Report on the Global Tobacco Epidemic, 2008—The MPOWER Package* emphasized tobacco-control strategies that include taxation, advertising bans, smoke-free policies on smoke-free environments, and enforcement of existing bans (WHO, 2008). WHO estimated that a 70% increase in tobacco price could prevent up to about 25% of all tobacco-related deaths worldwide (WHO, 2008). Tobacco companies often have offered coupons to offset the price increase, and the coupons circumvent the increase in price to the consumer (Chaloupka, 2002). Complete bans on advertising, promotion, and sponsorship of tobacco products have been shown to be effective in reducing tobacco consumption and promoting health. In addition to advertising bans, WHO recommends health warnings on tobacco packages, cessation programs, and treatment of tobacco dependence in all member states (WHO, 2008). According to WHO, resources for enforcement of smoke-free legislation and bans on advertising, promotion, and sponsorship of tobacco products require only small expenditures to yield major health benefits. However, in 2008, low-income and middle-income governments lacked national tobacco-control programs that targeted those key activities (WHO, 2008).

Even if there is not an active multiprong approach, the approval and implementation of a smoking ban at the local or state level usually involves much public debate, which itself increases public awareness of the health effects of smoking and secondhand smoke (IOM, 2007). Therefore, smoking behaviors often change before and beyond the restrictions put into place by legislation (for example, quitting or voluntary smoke-free workplace policies in anticipation of a ban, reduction in smoking in homes), and such changes would contribute to the magnitude of changes in health outcomes seen after the implementation of a smoking ban.

On an individual level, many smokers voluntarily refrain from smoking in some situations, for example, in their homes or cars or around their children. Among the possible reasons for that are increased awareness of health risks, wanting to be favorable role models, a desire for an odor-free environment, a change in social acceptability of smoking, or a desire to hide tobacco use (IOM, 2009). If those practices are adopted before a ban rather than following it, the apparent effect of the ban will be attenuated from the full effect and it can be difficult to assess how the ban itself changed exposure to secondhand smoke and to predict when a decrease in exposure might be expected to affect disease rates.

Comprehensive programs and voluntary actions could lead to larger decreases in smoking prevalence and a subsequent decrease in adverse health effects. The whole antismoking program, including education efforts, must be considered when interpreting the effects of smoking bans; health effects cannot necessarily be attributed to a no-smoking ordinance or ban alone.

Thus, in interpreting the results of studies that looked at a possible relationship between smoking bans and acute coronary events, caution must be taken not to attribute a decrease in adverse events solely to a reduction in secondhand smoke or to attribute a decrease in secondhand smoke solely to bans; other factors rather, contribute to the decreases. One major change that could occur with the implementation of smoking bans is a decrease in smoking—both through an increase in the number of people who quit smoking and through a decrease in the number of cigarettes smoked by smokers. As Figure 5-3 shows, the fall in per capita use of smoking preceded the common use of bans, which themselves resulted in decreased cigarette use and therefore less secondhand smoke exposure (HHS, 2000).

Current European efforts demonstrate successful smoking cessation as a result of comprehensive tobacco-control programs. An assessment of cross-sectional data from national health surveys in 18 European countries found quitting ratios[2] high (above 45%) in several countries, including Sweden, England, the Netherlands, Belgium, and France (Schaap et al., 2008). The study found a positive association between a national score on a tobacco-control scale and quitting ratios among all age–sex groups. Similarly, a prospective cohort survey in Ireland found steep declines in reported smoking in workplaces (48% reduction), restaurants (82%), and bars and pubs (93%) as a result of the implementation of comprehensive smoke-free workplace legislation in that country (Fong et al., 2006). The study reported that 46% of Irish smokers reported that they were more likely to quit smoking (although that is not the same as actually quitting) as a result of legislation enactment (Fong et al., 2006). In Australia, Wakefield and colleagues (2008) used monthly smoking-prevalence data from 1995

---

[2] Quitting ratios are calculated by dividing the numbers of total former smokers by the number of total ever-smokers.

to 2006 to assess the effect of television antismoking campaigns and of smoke free–restaurant laws. The study found that when the population was exposed about four times per month to antismoking advertising campaigns, smoking prevalence decreased by 0.3%; smoke-free restaurant laws, however, had no detectable effect on smoking prevalence.

In the United States, Fichtenberg and Glantz (2002) evaluated 26 studies of the effects of smoke-free workplaces in 2002; they found weak but significant inverse associations between completely smoke-free workplaces and smoking prevalence (3.8% reduction in prevalence; 95% confidence interval [CI], 2.8–4.7%) and daily cigarette consumption in continuing smokers (3.1 fewer cigarettes; 95% CI, 2.4–3.8). Messer et al. (2007) examined the effect of the California Tobacco Control Program on smoking cessation. The retrospective study assessed smoking history of 57,918 non-Hispanic white ever-smokers using data from the 1992–2002 Tobacco Use Supplements of the Current Populations Survey, monthly surveys conducted by the U.S. Census Bureau (Messer et al., 2007). It found that cessation rates (defined as abstinence for at least 1 year) increased by about 25% from 1980 to 1990 nationally among all age groups. Cessation rates averaged 3.4% per year in the 1990s. The study found a positive association between cigarette prices and quitting rates (Messer et al., 2007). Albers et al. (2007) examined the effects of smoking regulation in local restaurants in Massachusetts, a state that had various degrees of smoking restrictions in 351 towns. Adult smokers who had previously attempted to quit were about 3 times (odds ratio, 3.12; 95% CI, 1.51–6.44) more likely to attempt to quit in the 2 years after implementation of a smoking ban if they lived in towns with strong smoking regulations than if they did not, but no difference in smoking cessation was seen. The IOM report *Ending the Tobacco Problem: A Blueprint for the Nation* (IOM, 2007) concluded that comprehensive state tobacco programs can lead to substantial reductions in tobacco use. Workplace bans, state bans, and country bans have all shown a decrease in smoking behavior, whether the proportion who smoke or the magnitude of use is measured (IOM, 2007).

Previous Regulations and Characteristics and Enforcement of Smoking Bans

Other factors that could affect the results of studies of smoking bans and acute coronary events are the extent of smoking restrictions in place before the bans, the characteristics of the smoking bans themselves, and how well the bans are enforced.

As is evident in Table 5-1, smoking bans have been implemented at the city, county, and state level at various times in the United States. When the effect of a smoking ban on an adverse health effect is studied, the extent of reduction in the adverse effect depends in part on the extent of a restriction or partial ban that existed before the ban under study. For example, some locations had previously implemented partial bans, and some regions within the locations studied (for example, New York City and several other large counties in the New York state study) had previously implemented comprehensive bans (Juster et al., 2007). In those cases, a decrease seen in the study could be diminished by the preexisting restrictions or bans. Similarly, in studies that have comparison populations, partial restrictions in the control locations could affect the magnitude of differences seen.

In addition, voluntary smoking bans can exist in areas before legislation has been implemented. For example, many hotel chains, some restaurant chains, airlines and other mass transit systems, office buildings, health-care facilities, schools, and individually owned establishments instituted bans long before counties, cities, or states legislated bans. Categorizing a county as not having a smoking ban may fail to reflect the fact that the average smoker could spend a substantial amount of time in an occupational setting that prohibits smoking in and outside a building, could eat dinner in a restaurant that prohibits smoking, and could shop in stores that prohibit smoking. This is increasingly the case. In 1993, 46.5% of employees in the United States were covered by smoking restrictions; by 1998–1999, 69.3% were covered by smoking restrictions (Shopland et al., 2004). Such prohibitions have increased, so it is more difficult to attribute even temporal changes in tobacco use or exposure in a defined geographic area to the lack or presence of a smoking ordinance. That could contribute to an underestimate of the actual effect had there been no prior ban. In contrast, many bans have allowed smoking outside public buildings or more than some stated distance from entrances. Although it is possible that outside smoking could attenuate the benefits of a smoking ban, the concentrations of secondhand smoke in those areas, and the safety or hazardousness of such areas in human populations has yet to be evaluated.

If smoking bans decrease acute coronary events, the inclusiveness of a ban (for example, the types of buildings and establishments included and the number of exemptions allowed) would be expected to affect the magnitude of the decrease. Different bans can cover or exempt different types of establishments or locations (such as restaurants with bars, bowling alleys, bingo halls, and outdoor seating areas). In interpreting studies of smoking bans, especially in comparing results of different studies, it is important to consider the types and extent of different bans. In addition, if a ban is not complied with or enforced, changes in health effects would not be expected. For example, the Clean Indoor Air Act was enacted in 1985 by the Florida legislature, but enforcement usually depended on filing of complaints with the Department of Health (American Lung Association, 2009).

CONCLUSIONS

The issues raised in this chapter are relevant to the interpretation of the major studies that are the subject of this report. Recommendations for future studies are in Chapter 6.

- All the epidemiologic studies being reviewed should be evaluated in light of the amount of contextual data that are taken into account, including measurements both before and after bans and measurements comparing locales with and without bans.
- When study results are compared, it may be impossible to separate contextual factors associated with a ban—such as public comment periods, information announcing the ban, and notices about the impending changes—from the effect of the ban itself.
- The time from onset of a ban and concurrent activities to manifestation of disease can vary with the timing (and nature) of enforcement, and latency periods for cardiovascular incidents in people with different magnitudes of risk. Those factors, therefore, need to be considered in examining epidemiologic evidence.

REFERENCES

Albers, A. B., M. Siegel, D. M. Cheng, L. Biener, and N. A. Rigotti. 2007. Effect of smoking regulations in local restaurants on smokers' anti-smoking attitudes and quitting behaviours. *Tobacco Control* 16(2):101-106.

American Lung Association. 2009. *SLATI state information: Florida.* (Accessed April 1, 2009, from http://slati.lungusa.org/state-teml.asp?id=9.)

ANRF (American Nonsmokers' Rights Foundation). 2009. *Overview list—how many smoke-free laws?* (Accessed March 1, 2009, from http://www.no-smoke.org/goingsmokefree.php?id=519.)

Bayer, R., and J. Colgrove. 2002. Science, politics, and ideology in the campaign against environmental tobacco smoke. *American Journal of Public Health* 92(6):949-954.

CDC (Centers for Disease Control and Prevention). 2008. Disparities in secondhand smoke exposure—United States, 1988–1994 and 1999–2004 *MMWR—Morbidity & Mortality Weekly Report* 57(27):744-747.

Chaloupka, F., K. M. Cummings, C. P. Morley, and J. K. Horan. 2002. Tax, price and cigarette smoking: Evidence from the tobacco documents and implications for tobacco company marketing strategies. *Tobacco Control* 11(90001):i62-i72.

EPA (Environmental Protection Agency). 1992. *Respiratory health effects of passive smoking: Lung cancer and other disorders.* Washington, DC: Environmental Protection Agency.

Fichtenberg, C. M., and S. A. Glantz. 2002. Effect of smoke-free workplaces on smoking behaviour: Systematic review. *BMJ* 325(7357):188.

Fong, G. T., A. Hyland, R. Borland, D. Hammond, G. Hastings, A. McNeill, S. Anderson, K. M. Cummings, S. Allwright, M. Mulcahy, F. Howell, L. Clancy, M. E. Thompson, G. Connolly, and P. Driezen. 2006. Reductions in tobacco smoke pollution and increases in support for smoke-free public places following the implementation of comprehensive smoke-free workplace legislation in the Republic of Ireland: Findings from the ITC Ireland/UK survey. *Tobacco Control* 15 Suppl 3:iii51-iii58.

Garland, C., E. Barrett-Connor, L. Suarez, M. H. Criqui, and D. L. Wingard. 1985. Effects of passive smoking on ischemic heart disease mortality of nonsmokers. A prospective study. *American Journal of Epidemiology* 121(5):645-650.

HHS (U.S. Department of Health and Human Services). 1964. *Smoking and health: Report of the advisory committee of the surgeon general of the public health service*. Washington, DC: U.S. Department of Health, Education, and Welfare.

———. 1972. *The health consequences of smoking*. Atlanta, GA: U.S. Department of Health and Human Services, Centers for Disease Control and Prevention, National Center for Chronic Disease Prevention and Health Promotion, Office on Smoking and Health.

———. 1986. *The health consequences of involuntary smoking: A report of the surgeon general*. Atlanta, GA: U.S. Department of Health and Human Services, Centers for Disease Control and Prevention, National Center for Chronic Disease Prevention and Health Promotion, Office on Smoking and Health.

———. 2000. *Reducing tobacco use: A report of the surgeon general*. Atlanta, GA: U.S. Department of Health and Human Services, Centers for Disease Control and Prevention, National Center for Chronic Disease Prevention and Health Promotion, Office on Smoking and Health.

———. 2006. *The health consequences of involuntary exposure to tobacco smoke: A report of the surgeon general*. Atlanta, GA: U.S. Department of Health and Human Services, Centers for Disease Control and Prevention, National Coordinating Center for Health Promotion, National Center for Chronic Disease Prevention and Health Promotion, Office on Smoking and Health.

IARC (International Agency for Research on Cancer). 2008. *Methods for evaluating tobacco control policies*. Vol. 12, *IARC handbooks of cancer prevention in tobacco control*. Lyon, France: WHO.

IOM (Institute of Medicine). 2007. *Ending the tobacco problem: A blueprint for the nation*. Washington, DC: The National Academies Press.

———. 2009. *Combating tobacco in military and veteran populations*. Washington, DC: The National Academies Press.

Juster, H. R., B. R. Loomis, T. M. Hinman, M. C. Farrelly, A. Hyland, U. E. Bauer, and G. S. Birkhead. 2007. Declines in hospital admissions for acute myocardial infarction in New York state after implementation of a comprehensive smoking ban. *American Journal of Public Health* 97(11):2035-2039.

Koop, E. C. 1986. A society free of smoking by the year 2000? *World Health Forum* 7:225-231.

Messer, K., J. P. Pierce, S. H. Zhu, A. M. Hartman, W. K. Al-Delaimy, D. R. Trinidad, and E. A. Gilpin. 2007. The california tobacco control program's effect on adult smokers: (1) smoking cessation. *Tobacco Control* 16(2):85-90.

NRC (National Research Council). 1981. *Indoor air pollutants*. Washington, DC: National Academy Press.

———. 1986. *The airliner cabin environment: Air quality and safety*. Washington, DC: National Academy Press.

Schaap, M. M., A. E. Kunst, M. Leinsalu, E. Regidor, O. Ekholm, D. Dzurova, U. Helmert, J. Klumbiene, P. Santana, and J. P. Mackenbach. 2008. Effect of nationwide tobacco control policies on smoking cessation in high and low educated groups in 18 European countries. *Tobacco Control* 17(4):248-255.

Shopland, D. R., C. M. Anderson, D. M. Burns, and K. K. Gerlach. 2004. Disparities in smoke-free workplace policies among food service workers. *Journal of Occupational & Environmental Medicine* 46:347-356.

Wakefield, M. A., S. Durkin, M. J. Spittal, M. Siahpush, M. Scollo, J. A. Simpson, S. Chapman, V. White, and D. Hill. 2008. Impact of tobacco control policies and mass media campaigns on monthly adult smoking prevalence. *American Journal of Public Health* 98(8):1443-1450.

WHO (World Health Organization). 2005. *WHO framework convention on tobacco control.*

———. 2007. *Protection from exposure to second-hand tobacco smoke: Policy recommendations.* Geneva: World Health Organization.

———. 2008. *WHO report on the global tobacco epidemic, 2008: The MPOWER package.* Geneva: World Health Organization.

———. 2009. *Parties to the WHO framework convention on tobacco control.* (Accessed March 31, 2009, from http://www.who.int/fctc/signatories_parties/en/index.html.) Geneva: World Health Organization.

6

Overview of Key Studies of the Effects of Smoking Bans on Acute Coronary Events

In this chapter, the committee discusses key studies, and 11 publications from those studies, of the effects of smoking bans on acute coronary events. The articles reviewed in this chapter address two of the associations that the committee is evaluating:

- The association between secondhand-smoke exposure and acute coronary events (Questions 2, 3, and 5, see Box 1-1).
- The association between smoking bans and acute coronary events (Questions 4, 5, 6, 7, and 8, see Box 1-1).

Eleven publications deal with studies that looked at the effects of smoking bans in eight natural experiments: three studies in overlapping regions of Italy (Barone-Adesi et al., 2006; Cesaroni et al., 2008; Vasselli et al., 2008); one study in Pueblo, Colorado, after 18 months of followup (Bartecchi et al., 2006) and after 3 years of followup (CDC, 2009); and one study each in Helena, Montana (Sargent et al., 2004), Monroe County, Indiana (Seo and Torabi, 2007), Bowling Green, Ohio (Khuder et al., 2007), New York state (Juster et al., 2007), Saskatoon, Canada (Lemstra et al., 2008), and Scotland (Pell et al., 2008). The legislation in Bowling Green, Ohio, allowed smoking in some restaurants and bars; it called for a smoking restriction rather than a smoking ban. The studies examined changes in heart-attack rates, or acute myocardial infarctions (acute MIs) after the implementation of the bans (and one restriction) and were not designed to answer questions about the association between exposure to secondhand smoke and cardiovascular disease. Most of the studies did not measure individual exposures to secondhand smoke or the smoking status of individuals; thus, they were designed to evaluate the association between smoking bans and acute MIs, not the effects of secondhand-smoke exposure. The publications on the smoking bans in Monroe County, Indiana, and Scotland, however, contain data on smoking status and results of analyses only in nonsmokers; these two studies were designed to assess the association between secondhand-smoke exposure and acute MIs.

The committee discusses the studies below, including information on the smoking bans and restriction in the different locations, available information on secondhand-smoke exposure, study designs, and study results. Publications that examine the effect of the same smoking ban are discussed together; the most comprehensive or recent publication is discussed first. The different smoking bans are discussed in order by earliest publication date. Details of the smoking bans and restriction in the different regions are presented in Table 6-1; available information on the effect of the bans on potential secondhand smoke exposure—including data on enforcement and compliance, air monitoring, and biomonitoring—is presented in Table 6-2; and details of the study designs and published results are presented in Table 6-3.

HELENA, MONTANA

Smoking Ban and Exposure Information

Helena, Montana, enacted and enforced legislation requiring smoke-free workplaces and public places for the period June 5–December 3, 2002. The legislation banned smoking in restaurants, bars, and other workplaces and protected an estimated population of 28,726 (ANRF, 2009).

One publication examined the relationship between the Helena smoking ban and acute coronary events (Sargent et al., 2004). The committee did not identify any studies reporting air monitoring or biomonitoring for potential secondhand-smoke exposure in Helena before and after the ban compared with during the ban. Regarding compliance, Sargent et al. (2004) state that "the city–county health department reported that all but two businesses complied" with the ordinance, citing a letter to the editor of the *Helena Independent Review*. The study provided information directly related to the association between smoking bans and acute coronary events.

Published Results on Acute Coronary Events

Sargent et al. (2004) studied the effect of the smoking-ban legislation on hospital admissions for acute MI in Helena, Montana. The study

TABLE 6-1 Characteristics of Smoking Bans Assessed in Key Surveillance Studies

Location	References[a]	Effective Date	Restaurants	Bars	Workplaces	Other
Helena, Montana[b]	Sargent et al., 2004	6/05/2002	✓	✓	✓	Gaming establishments
Italy	Barone-Adesi, 2006; Cesaroni et al., 2008; Vasselli et al., 2008	1/10/2005	✓	✓	✓	Retail shops, cafés, discotheques
Pueblo, Colorado	Bartecchi et al., 2006; CDC, 2009	7/01/2003	✓	✓	✓	✓
Monroe County, Indiana	Seo and Torabi, 2007	8/01/2003	✓	✓ (effective 1/1/2005)	✓	
Bowling Green, Ohio	Khuder et al., 2007	03/2002	✓ (except isolated bar, isolated smoking area)	Bars at owner discretion	✓	Bowling alleys at owner discretion
New York state[c]	Juster et al., 2007	7/24/2003	✓	✓	✓	✓
Saskatoon, Canada	Lemstra et al., 2008	7/01/2004	✓	✓	✓	✓
Scotland[d]	Pell et al., 2008	03/2006	✓	✓	✓	✓

[a] Data from cited references unless otherwise stated.
[b] Information on smoking-ban locations also from helenair.com (http://www.helenair.com/articles/2002/09/25/stories/helena/1a2.txt), accessed July 2009.
[c] A number of local smoking bans and restrictions were in place in New York state before the implementation of the statewide ban.
[d] Exceptions included "residential accommodation and designated room in hotels, care homes, hospices, and psychiatric units" (Haw and Gruer, 2007).

TABLE 6-2 Potential Secondhand-Smoke Exposure Reductions in Key Publications[a]

Location of Ban (Implementation Date)	Smoking Ban Details
Helena, Montana (June 5, 2002; rescinded December 3, 2002)	No prior ban mentioned Legislation to require smoke-free workplaces and public places; suspended as a result of litigation after about 6 months Smoking banned in restaurants, bars, other workplaces
Italy (January 10, 2005)	Ban on smoking in all indoor public places, including offices, retail shops, cafes, bars, restaurants, discotheques in Italy; provision for smoking rooms
Pueblo, Colorado (July 1, 2003)	Ban prohibiting smoking in workplaces, all public buildings (including restaurants, bars, bowling alleys, other business establishments) within city limits
Monroe County, Indiana (August 1, 2003; extended to bars January 1, 2005)	Ban in all restaurants, retail stores, workplaces; extended to previously exempt bars and clubs January 1, 2005
Bowling Green, Ohio (March 2002)	Ban in public places except bars, restaurants with bars if bars are isolated with separate smoking areas; bars, bowling alleys could allow smoking at owners' discretion

Information on Decreased Exposure or Compliance

No air monitoring, but key publication (Sargent et al., 2004) refers to newspaper letter to editor that
reports that City–County Health Department reported that all but two businesses complied

No information in key publications looking at acute MI (Barone-Adesi et al., 2006; Cesaroni et al., 2008)

Survey indicated that almost 90% of surveyed population (selected locations in Italy) perceived that ban
was observed in bars, restaurants; 70% in workplaces (Gallus et al., 2006)

Letter to editor presented data on nicotine vapor phase in pubs, discos in Florence before, after
implementation of ban; pre-implementation median, 138.9 $\mu g/m^3$ (range, 33.0–276.5 $\mu g/m^3$),
postimplementation median, 4.5 $\mu g/m^3$ (range, 1.7–8.7 $\mu g/m^3$)—decreased to average of 3.2% of the
pre-ban concentrations (Gorini et al., 2005)

Fine, ultrafine particles before and after implementation in 40 establishments in Rome, urinary cotinine
in nonsmoking employees (Valente et al., 2007):

Average PM$_{2.5}$: decreased from 119.3 $\mu g/m^3$ to 38.2 $\mu g/m^3$ (p < 0.005), 43.3 $\mu g/m^3$ (p < 0.01) 2–3
months, 11–12 months after implementation, respectively

Average ultrafine particles: decreased but not to as great an extent—from 76,956 particles/cm^3 to
38,079 particles/cm^3 (p < 0.0001), 51,692 particles/cm^3 (p < 0.01) 2–3 months, 11–12 months after
implementation, respectively

Average urinary cotinine: decreased from 17.8 ng/mL (95% CI, 14–21.6 ng/mL) to 5.5 ng/mL (95% CI,
3.8–7.2), 3.7 ng/mL (95% CI, 1.8–5.6 ng/mL) 2–3 months, 11–12 months after implementation,
respectively

No information on decreased concentrations of SHS components, but enforcement officials strongly
supported ban with strict fines and ban was implemented after vote indicating public support for it
(Bartecchi et al., 2006; CDC, 2009)

No information on decreased concentrations of SHS components or compliance (Seo and Torabi, 2007)

No information on concentrations of SHS components or compliance provided in key health publication
(Khuder et al., 2007)

Concentrations of SHS-related compounds (including nicotine, 3-ethenylpyridine, total RSP, RSP based
on Solanesol, UVPM, FPM) in four restaurants, one smoke-free and one smoking (that is, with bar)
each in Toledo, Bowling Green, Ohio; data from previous study were compared with data from
average concentrations in two cities combined; analyses indicated that concentrations of SHS-
related contaminants did not change after smoking restrictions, but concentrations were lower in
nonsmoking restaurants than restaurants that allow smoking in separate areas (Akbar-Khanzadeh et
al., 2004)

Continued

TABLE 6-2 Continued

Location of Ban (Implementation Date)	Smoking Ban Details
New York state (July 24, 2003)	New York's Clean Indoor Air Act is 100% statewide ban on smoking in all workplaces, including restaurants, bars, gaming establishments, with limited exceptions Statewide smoking restrictions (limiting or prohibiting smoking in some public places, such as schools, hospitals, public buildings, retail stores) had been implemented in 1989 Previously, smoking bans of various levels implemented at city or county level in some parts of state, including ban in workplaces—such as restaurants, bars—in New York City, several other large jurisdictions State law does not pre-empt passage of local laws
Saskatoon, Canada (July 1, 2004)	Smoking ban in city of Saskatoon prohibiting smoking in any enclosed public space open to public or to which public is customarily admitted or invited; smoking also prohibited in outdoor seating areas for restaurants, licensed premises Previously, smoking prohibited in government buildings As of January 1, 2005, 100% smoke-free law in all public places, workplaces, including restaurants, bars, bingo halls, bowling alleys, casinos in Saskatchewan; local municipalities have right to enact smoke-free air regulations
Scotland (March 2006)	Smoking prohibited in all enclosed public places, workplaces throughout Scotland, including bars, pubs, restaurants, cafes; exceptions included residential accommodations, designated rooms in hotels, care homes, hospices, psychiatric units

Abbreviations: CI, confidence interval; FPM, fluorescent particulate matter; MI, myocardial infarction; NYATS, New York Adult Tobacco Survey; PM, particulate matter; RSP, respirable suspended particulate matter; SHS, secondhand smoke; UVPM, respirable suspended ultraviolet particulate matter.

[a] This table contains information on the concentration of airborne tracers or biomarkers of secondhand smoke in locations of key surveillance studies. The locations are presented in the order they are presented in the text.

Information on Decreased Exposure or Compliance

No information in key study (Juster et al., 2007), but authors cite NYATS study showing decrease in
   salivary cotinine from 0.078 ng/mL (range, 0.054–0.111 ng/mL) to 0.041 ng/mL (range, 0.036–0.047
   ng/mL) in sample of New York state adults after implementation of ban (CDC, 2007)
NYATS (CDC, 2007) also asked about exposures to SHS; number of respondents reporting exposure to
   SHS in restaurants, bars decreased, but not significantly in workplaces, after implementation of ban:
   In Restaurants: from 19.8% (95% CI, 15.6–24.1%) reporting exposure to 3.1% (95% CI,
      2.0–4.2%) 9–10 months after ban
   In Bars: from 52.4% (95% CI, 41.5–63.4%) reporting exposure to 13.4% (95% CI, 9.5–17.3%) 10
      months after ban
   In Workplaces: from 13.6% (95% CI, 8.1–19.1%) reporting exposure to 7.6% (95% CI, 5.1–10.2%)
      9–10 months after ban
Hospitality venues in western New York before, after 2003 ban: average $PM_{2.5}$ concentration decreased
   from 324 $\mu g/m^3$ before implementation of ban to 25 $\mu g/m^3$ after ($p < 0.001$) (CDC, 2004)
Juster et al. (2007) cite report by Research Triangle Institute, International (RTI International, 2004)
   that showed that 93% of restaurants, bars, bowling facilities were in compliance in year after
   implementation
Business compliance with ban measured by reviewing warnings, tickets issued by public-health inspectors
   to eligible businesses; of 924 eligible establishments, 914 were inspected within first 6 months of
   ban; of 914, only 13 had to be issued noncompliance warning (for not posting signs or not removing
   ashtrays); one ticket was issued on reinspection (Lemstra et al., 2008)

Self-reported survey provided information about exposure to SHS; number of people who had never
   smoked reporting no exposure to smoke increased (from 57 to 78%; $p < 0.001$); individual serum
   cotinine measurements taken; geometric mean in never smokers decreased from 0.68 to 0.56 ng/mL
   ($p < 0.001$) after legislation enacted; similar data seen in former smokers (Pell et al., 2008)
Before ban, $PM_{2.5}$ concentrations ranged from 8 to 902 $\mu g/m^3$ (average, 246 $\mu g/m^3$); after implementation
   of ban, concentrations ranged from 6 to 104 $\mu g/m^3$ (average, 20 $\mu g/m^3$) (Semple et al., 2007a)
In nonsmokers, geometric mean cotinine concentration decreased by more than 39%, from 0.43 to 0.26
   ng/mL after implementation of ban ($p < 0.001$) (Haw and Gruer, 2007)
In nonsmokers, geometric mean salivary cotinine concentration decreased from 2.9 ng/mL before ban to
   0.7 ng/mL 2 months after and to 0.4 ng/mL 1 year after in 301 bar workers (Semple et al., 2007b)
Serum cotinine concentrations in bar workers in Dundee and Perth, Scotland, decreased from 5.15 ng/mL
   before ban to 3.22 ng/mL 1 month after (reduction of 1.93 ng/mL; 95% CI, 1.03–2.83 ng/mL; $p <$
   0.001) and to 2.93 ng/mL 2 months after (reduction of 2.22 ng/mL; 95% CI, 1.34–3.10 ng/mL; $p <$
   0.001) (Menzies et al., 2006)

population included consecutive patients admitted to St. Peter's Community Hospital with a primary or secondary diagnosis of acute MI (*International Classification of Diseases, Revision 9 [ICD-9]* 410.xx) during the period December 1997–November 2003. Selection of patients to include in the study was based on a review of paper and electronic medical records and billing records for June–November (the months during which the ban was in effect in 2002) of 1998–2003. Data were included if a patient had primary or secondary acute MI, on the basis of the attending physician's diagnosis of acute MI, the onset of symptoms occurred in the study area, and there was no recent procedure that could have precipitated the acute MI. If a patient had a secondary diagnosis of acute MI, patient information was included only if there was increased troponin I concentration or creatine phosphokinase activity at admission or within 24 h of admission and there was no recent precipitating procedure. The authors compared the number of hospital admissions during the months when the smoking ban was in effect in 2002 with the average number of admissions during the same months in the 4 years before and 1 year after the ban. A total of 304 admissions met the inclusion criteria.

The authors found a statistically significant reduction in the number of hospital admissions during the period when the smoking ban was in effect, from an average of 40 in June–November in the years before and after the ban was in place (1998–2001 and 2003) to a total of 24 admissions in the same months of 2002, when the smoking ban was in effect (16 fewer admissions; 95% confidence interval [CI], 0.3 to 31.7). The authors noted a nonsignificant *increase* of 5.6 additional events in hospital admissions in the unincorporated area surrounding Helena used as a control during the same study period.

An advantage of the study design is that the suspension of enforcement of the smoking ban allowed a "cross-over comparison" of incidence before, during, and after the ban and the presence of a control community. Study limitations included the small population, the reliance on historical controls, and the lack of direct exposure information or information on individual smoking status. The study did not account for the potential effect of the ban on primary smokers (for example, if smokers quit), so direct conclusions can be drawn only on the effect of the smoking ban and associated activities, not on the effect of secondhand-smoke exposure. The study also lacked controls for other cardiovascular risk factors. With regard to the outcome information, collection of data only from records of those who reached the hospital could miss some fatal cases of acute MI, and the criteria for diagnosing acute MI changed during the study period as the hospital began requiring a troponin I concentration for diagnosis. The authors did, however, conduct a regression analysis to test whether troponin I concentration was an important factor in the analysis and found that it did not affect the study results.

ITALY

Smoking Ban and Exposure Information

On January 10, 2005, Italy implemented a nationwide smoking ban in all indoor public places, including offices, retail shops, cafés, bars, restaurants, and discotheques. Smoking was not banned in private houses or specifically equipped public areas (for example, the law had requirements for exempted areas, including ventilation systems that create negative pressure and a requirement for doors) (Vasselli et al., 2008).

Although no exposure data are available on the specific populations, some general compliance and monitoring data are available from before and after implementation of the ban. Gallus et al. (2006) found that of 3,114 people ages 15 years or older who were surveyed in Italy, almost 90% perceived that the ban was observed in bars, and 70% had that perception for workplaces. As reported by Gorini et al. (2005) in a letter to a journal editor, the median concentration of nicotine in the vapor phase of samples from four pubs and three discotheques in Florence decreased to an average of 3.2% of the pre-ban median: from 138.9 $\mu g/m^3$ (range, 33.0–276.5 $\mu g/m^3$) to 4.5 $\mu g/m^3$ (range, 1.7–8.7 $\mu g/m^3$). Valente et al. (2007) measured fine and ultrafine particles in 40 establishments in Rome and urinary cotinine in nonsmoking employees of the establishments before and after implementation of the ban. The average concentration of $PM_{2.5}$ particles (particles smaller than 2.5 μm in aerodynamic diameter) decreased from 119.3 $\mu g/m^3$ before the ban to 38.2 $\mu g/m^3$ ($p < 0.005$) 2–3 months after implementation and to 43.3 $\mu g/m^3$ ($p < 0.01$) 11–12 months after implementation. The average concentration of ultrafine particles also decreased but to a smaller extent, from 76,956 particles/cm^3 before the ban to 38,079 particles/cm^3 ($p < 0.0001$) and 51,692 particles/cm^3 ($p < 0.01$) 2–3 months and 11–12 months after implementation, respectively. Urinary cotinine in the employees decreased from an average of 17.8 ng/mL (95% CI, 14–21.6 ng/mL) before the ban to 5.5 ng/mL (95% CI, 3.8–7.2 ng/mL) and 3.7 ng/mL (95% CI, 1.8–5.6 ng/mL) 2–3 months and 11–12 months after implementation, respectively. Those data indicate that the smoking ban resulted in a decrease in exposure to secondhand smoke.

Published Results on Acute Coronary Events

Three publications report on acute coronary events after implementation of the Italian smoking ban (Barone-Adesi et al., 2006; Cesaroni et

TABLE 6-3 Summary of Results of Key Publications (Studies Listed by Smoking-Ban Region in Order of Publication)

Publication (Region)	Study Design and Duration	Selection of Patients
Helena, Montana		
Sargent et al., 2004 (Helena, Montana)	Retrospective based on hospital records; 6 months of ban, 11 months after ban compared with same months of 5 years before ban	Patients 18 years old and older admitted to St. Peter's Community Hospital for primary or secondary diagnosis of acute MI (*ICD-9* 410. xx) Selection criteria: onset of symptoms in study area, no recent procedure that could have precipitated acute MI, primary diagnosis of acute MI or secondary diagnosis with chemical evidence of acute MI at time of admission (cTn or creatine phosphokinase) Control population: county residents who lived outside city boundaries
Italy		
Vasselli et al., 2008 (four regions in Italy: Piedmont, Friuli–Venezia–Giulia, Latium, Campania)	Retrospective based on hospital discharge registry; study period January 10–March 10, 2001–2005; compared 2 months after ban with same 2 months of 4 years before ban	Patients in public, private hospitals with primary discharge diagnosis of acute MI, 40–64 years old; hospital data from National Hospital Discharge Registry (2001, 2002, 2003), which is based on regional data, or from regional hospital discharge registries for years not previously incorporated into national registry (2004, 2005)

Results	Statistical Analysis	Comments
Total of 304 cases met selection criteria; 24 cases in Helena during ban; 18 cases outside Helena during ban Average monthly admissions declined from 40 to 24 (16 fewer admissions; 95% CI, 0.3–31.7) during same months in years before and after implementation of ban Nonsignificant increase of 5.6 in number of acute MI admissions from outside Helena during same period	Mean comparisons before, after ban implementation, and between areas with Poisson distribution for counts	No information on individual smoking status; no measures of individual SHS exposure Small population Advantage of having data before ban, during ban, after rescinding of ban Criteria for diagnosing acute MI changed during study period
Cases: 2001, 1,309; 2002, 1,408; 2003, 1,511; 2004, 1,589; 2005, 1,488 Total of all four regions: rates increased linearly from 2001 to 2004, decreased by 6.4% from 2004 to 2005 Regional level: rates less linear than total of all four regions; rates increased or unchanged from 2001 to 2004; rates decreased from 2004 to 2005 (significantly in Piedmont, Latium, Campania) Total of all four regions, observed 2005 versus expected based on linear regression: risk reduction 13.1% (age-standardized risk ratio, 0.86; 95% CI, 0.83–0.92) Significant decrease from expected numbers in 2005 in men but not women 45–49 years old but not other age ranges, all regions except Friuli–Venezia–Giulia	Comparison of age-standardized rates, subgroup comparisons for sex, age, region separately	No information on individual smoking status; no measures of individual SHS exposure Limited study duration; looked only at effects 2 months after implementation of; population was less than 30% of Italy Rates standardized by overall total, age, region, sex

Continued

TABLE 6-3 Continued

Publication (Region)	Study Design and Duration	Selection of Patients
Barone-Adesi, 2006 (Piedmont region, northern Italy)	Retrospective based on records from regional hospital discharge registry; 5 pre-ban months studied, ending 6 months before implementation; 6 months after implementation of ban studied, starting at beginning of ban	Hospital admissions with primary diagnosis of acute MI (*ICD-9* 401), hospital deaths due to acute MI
Cesaroni et al., 2008 (Rome, Italy)	Retrospective based on hospital discharge registry, death registry; January 1, 2000–December 31, 2005; followup just under 12 months after implementation	Cases identified from all hospitalizations of city residents at public, private hospitals in Rome, regional register that tracks all causes of death Cases defined as principal diagnosis of acute MI (*ICD-9-CM* 410) or other acute, subacute forms of ischemic heart disease (*ICD-9-CM* 411), secondary diagnosis of acute MI with principal diagnosis indicating acute MI complications (for example, 427.1, paroxysmal ventricular tachycardia; 427.41, ventricular fibrillation)
Pueblo, Colorado CDC, 2009 (Pueblo, Colorado)	Retrospective based on hospital admission data; duration 1.5 years before, 1.5 and 3.0 years after implementation of smoke-free ordinance	All patients with primary diagnosis of acute MI (*ICD-9* 401.xx) admitted to Parkview Medical Center or St. Mary-Corwin Medical Center January 1, 2002–June 30, 2006 Assessed number of fatal acute MIs in residents in Pueblo city limits (based on residential ZIP codes) around time smoke-free ordinance was passed Control populations in Pueblo County but outside city limits, El Paso County Analyzed data after implementation of smoking ban (January 2005–June 30, 2006; phase II after implementation) compared with 1.5 years before implementation (January 2002–June 2003), 0–1.5 years after implementation (July 2003–December 2004; phase I after implementation; previously analyzed in Bartecchi et al., 2006)

Results	Statistical Analysis	Comments
922 cases before implementation of ban; 832 cases after Rates of admission for acute MI decreased in people under 60 years old (RR, 0.89; 95% CI, 0.81–0.98) but not in those over 60 years old; decrease statistically significant in men, women under 60 years old	Comparison of age-standardized incidence rates; subgroup analysis by sex, age; linear dose–response analysis for effects of smoking	No information on individual smoking status; no measures of individual SHS exposure No data on potential confounders collected
14,075 acute coronary events documented during study period Age-standardized rates of annual acute coronary events decreased after implementation of ban in 35- to 64-year-olds (RR, 0.89; 95% CI, 0.85–0.93), 65- to 74-year-olds (RR, 0.92; 95% CI, 0.88–0.97) but not those over 74 years old	Age-standardized rates; Poisson regression applied to annual data with adjustment for sex, age, SES	No information on individual smoking status; no measures of individual SHS exposure Potential confounders—such as particulate-matter air pollution, temperature, influenza epidemics, time trends, total hospitalization rates—taken into account Data on cigarette sales in Rome, population smoking habits in Rome region included
Total of 1,559 cases for phase II: 237 in Pueblo city; 92 in Pueblo County (not in city); 1,230 in El Paso County City of Pueblo: phase II relative to phase I, RR = 0.81 (95% CI, 0.67–0.96); phase II relative to pre-implementation, 0.59 (95% CI, 0.49–0.70) Pueblo County: phase II relative to phase I, 1.21 (95% CI, 0.80–1.62); phase II relative to pre-implementation, 1.03 (95% CI, 0.68–1.39) El Paso County: phase II relative to phase I, 0.99 (95% CI, 0.91–1.08); phase II relative to pre-implementation, 0.95 (95% CI, 0.87–1.03)	Chi-square test to compare rates over time	No information on individual smoking status; no measures of individual SHS exposure Excluded secondary acute MI diagnoses, all acute MI patients transferred from outside facilities, residents with ZIP codes outside Pueblo County Adjustment of acute MI rates for season, air pollution—but not directly for inclusion of control community (El Paso County), where air-pollution fluctuations are similar—reduced possibility of variability

Continued

TABLE 6-3 Continued

Publication (Region)	Study Design and Duration	Selection of Patients
Bartecchi et al., 2006 (Pueblo, Colorado)	Same as CDC (2009) but only after 1.5 years of followup	Same as CDC (2009) but data collected only through December 2004
Monroe County, Indiana Seo and Torabi, 2007 (Monroe County, Indiana)	Retrospective based on records; study period August 1, 2001–May 31, 2005, that is, 22 months before enforcement and 22 months after	Primary, secondary diagnosis of acute MI (*ICD-9-CM* 410.xx) admitted to Bloomington Hospital, Ball Memorial Hospital; no past cardiac procedure or comorbidity that could have precipitated acute MI; chemical evidence of event onset of symptoms in study location Delaware County selected as control county on basis of similar urban population rates, income, cancer mortality

Results	Statistical Analysis	Comments
<u>Total of 2,794 patients</u>: 690 in Pueblo city; 165 in Pueblo County (not in city); 1,939 in El Paso County Acute MI hospitalizations decreased in Pueblo city residents after ordinance (RR, 0.73; 95% CI, 0.63–0.85) No significant changes in acute MI rates in Pueblo County residents (RR, 0.85; 95% CI, 0.63–1.16), El Paso County residents (RR, 0.97; 95% CI, 0.89–1.06) Acute MI rate decrease in Pueblo residents compared with El Paso County (p < 0.001)	Chi-square test to compare sex differences across locale; ANOVA to test mean age equality; Tukey multiple-comparison procedure to compare age pairs; Poisson regression on monthly data to model seasonality with two harmonics	In addition to comments on CDC (2009), only 1.5 years of follow-up
Cases: Monroe County, 22; Delaware County, 34 Monroe County: significant decrease in number of nonsmoking-patient admissions for acute MI (admissions decreased from 17 to 5; 95% CI, 2.81–21.19) from period 1 (August 2001–May 2003, before smoking ban) to period 2 (August 2003–May 2005, smoking ban in effect) Delaware County (control): nonsignificant decrease in number of nonsmoking-patient admissions (admissions decreased from 18 to 16; 95% CI, decrease of 9.43–13.43) from period 1 to period 2 Significant difference in nonsmoking-patient admissions between two counties in period 2 (5 Monroe County, 16 Delaware County)	Comparison of counts before, after with Poisson regression	Included only nonsmoking patients; smoking status based on patient charts No measures of individual SHS exposure Admission charts were reviewed Data collected on admission date, smoking status, comorbidity, whether past cardiac procedure could have precipitated acute MI, laboratory values, including troponin I concentrations or creatine phophokinase Excluded people with history of past cardiac events, hypertension, high cholesterol No information on age Excluded 2 months from analysis (June 1, 2003–July 31, 2003) to control for season variation

Continued

TABLE 6-3 Continued

Publication (Region)	Study Design and Duration	Selection of Patients
Bowling Green, Ohio Khuder et al., 2007 (Bowling Green, Ohio)	Retrospective based on hospital discharge records in 1999–2005; assessment from October 2002 to 39 months after ordinance went into effect (ordinance in effect in March 2002)	Admission rates for adults (over 18 years old) with primary diagnosis of coronary events (angina, heart failure, atherosclerosis, MI; ICD-9 410–413, 428); residents of Bowling Green, Ohio, and control city (Kent, Ohio) 2000 census population data used as denominator for rates
New York state Juster et al., 2007 (New York state)	Retrospective based on hospital discharge records; estimates of admissions calculated statistically; data for January 1995–December 2004 (17 months after statewide ban)	Monthly hospital admissions associated with acute MI (ICD-9-CM 410.0–410.99), stroke (ICD-9-CM 430.00–438.99), persons 35 years old and older Data extracted for all 62 New York counties

Results	Statistical Analysis	Comments
3,235 acute coronary syndrome cases before ban; 2,684 after ban implementation 36/10,000 people in 2002, 22/10,000 in 2003, 19/10,000 in first half of 2005 39% decrease (95% CI, 33–45%) in 2002 47% decrease (95% CI, 41–55%) in data after 3 years Significant decrease in trend (measure of change in series level, $\omega = -1.69$; $p = 0.04$) in monthly series rates 7 months after full implementation and enforcement (November 2002) Significant trend not seen in Kent No decrease seen after 6 months	Age-standardized rates; rate comparison with Mantel–Haenszel chi-square tests; monthly data analyzed with ARIMA time-series analysis, change in level at 6 months after implementation	No significant difference in non-smoking-related admissions in either Bowling Green or Kent No information on individual smoking status; no measures of individual SHS exposure
Annual averages over 10-year period: 46,000 admissions for acute MI, more than 58,000 admissions for stroke No change in trend line for hospital admissions for acute MI with implementation of 2003 statewide ban Estimated 3,813 (8%) fewer hospital admissions for acute MI than would be expected in absence of state smoking ban in 2004 Estimated 19% decline in admissions would have been associated with the comprehensive state law if large number of jurisdictions in state had not already had ordinances	Multiple linear regression for interrupted time series to analyze monthly age-, sex-adjusted county rates	No information on individual smoking status; no measures of individual SHS exposure Excluded restrictions applied only to municipal buildings New York County smoking restrictions categorized as comprehensive or moderate[a]

Continued

TABLE 6-3 Continued

Publication (Region)	Study Design and Duration	Selection of Patients
Saskatoon, Canada		
Lemstra et al., 2008 (Saskatoon, Canada)	Retrospective based on hospital discharge records; compared first full year of public smoking ban (July 1, 2004–June 30, 2005) compared with previous 4 years (July 1, 2000–June 30, 2004)	Diagnosis of acute MI (*ICD-410.xx*); age-standardized incidence of acute MI per 100,000 people
Scotland		
Pell et al., 2008 (Scotland)	Prospective; 10 months before (June 2005–March 2006), 10 months after (June 2006–March 2007) implementation of smoking ban	All patients admitted to nine hospitals with acute coronary syndrome (defined as detectable cTn after emergency admission for chest pain)

Abbreviations: CI, confidence interval; cTn, cardiac troponin; *ICD-9-CM, International Classification of Diseases, Revision 9, Clinical Modification*; MI, myocardial infarction; RR, relative risk; SES, socioeconomic status; SHS, secondhand smoke.

al., 2008; Vasselli et al., 2008) and provide information directly related to the association between smoking bans and acute coronary events. All three publications include data on acute coronary events through 2005, but Vasselli et al. (2008) analyzed data from the largest number of regions, which included the regions analyzed in the other two publications.

Vasselli et al. (2008) compared admissions for acute MI in the 2 months (January 10–March 10, 2005) after the January 10, 2005, implementation of the ban on smoking in all indoor public places in Italy with admissions in the same 2-month periods in 2001–2004. Data were collected from the National Hospital Discharge Registry and from the regional hospital discharge registries in four Italian regions that make up 28% of the Italian population, which had data available on the relevant times and were willing

Results	Statistical Analysis	Comments
1,689 cases of acute MI observed during 5-year study period Age-standardized incidence of acute MI decreased from 176.1 cases/100,000 to 152.4 cases/100,000 after implementation of public smoking ban (13%; rate ratio, 0.87; 95% CI, 0.84–0.90) Smoking prevalence decreased from 24.1 to 18.2% in Saskatoon from 2003 to 2005 (unchanged in Saskatchewan at 23.8%; smaller reduction in Canada overall from 22.9 to 21.3%)	Comparison of age-standardized incidence rates	No information on individual smoking status; no measures of individual SHS exposure No control city; therefore, no comparative time trends assessed Random telephone survey of 1,255 Saskatoon adult residents conducted 1 year after implementation of ban to collect information on smoking behavior and attitudes toward ban
Admissions for acute coronary syndrome decreased by 17% (95% CI, 16–18%) after implementation of ban; greatest reduction in admissions observed in nonsmokers	Compared binary, ordinal data with chi-square test; subgroup analyses by sex, age; two-sample t-test, log transformation on cotinine concentrations	Detailed information on smoking, exposure to SHS from questionnaires, biochemical assays Self-reported smoking status Serum cotinine concentrations used to categorize smoking status, SHS exposure

[a] Comprehensive laws prohibit smoking in all worksites, including restaurants, bars, and hospitality venues with few or no exemptions; moderate laws restrict smoking in most worksites but provide little or no protection in hospitality venues.

to participate in the study: Piedmont, Friuli–Venezia–Giulia, Latium, and Campania.

The study population included residents of the four areas who were 40–64 years old and who had been admitted to a hospital in the regions during the study months for acute events that had a primary discharge diagnosis of acute MI (*ICD-9* 410.xx). A total of 7,305 cases of acute MI were reported in the publication over the 4-year period. Only new events were considered; specifically, events that occurred less than 28 days after a first hospital admission for acute MI were excluded. The authors stated, "The mean age was chosen because the risk of myocardial infarction is high among persons over 64 years and low among those under 40 years. The 40–64 year category represents a group with a higher probability of being employed and in good health, and thereby having a higher attributable risk of acute MI due to passive smoke in the workplace and thus more sensitive to acute changes in exposure occurring as a result of the new law." Admission rates and age-standardized admission rates were calculated for the same period before and after implementation of the ban by using the European standard population as the reference population. Linear regression was used to estimate expected values and rates of admission; differences between expected and observed values were analyzed overall and by sex, age, and region.

From January 10 to March 10, 2001, 2002, 2003, 2004, and 2005, totals of 1,309, 1,408, 1,511, 1,589, and 1,488 acute coronary events, respectively, occurred in the four Italian regions. The corresponding age-standardized rates are 24.7, 26.4, 28.2, 29.5, and 27.2 per 100,000 person-years, respectively. The data suggest that the absolute numbers and rates of events increased each year from 2001 through 2004 and then decreased in 2005, although the rate was higher in 2005 than 2001 and 2002. The trend of an increase from 2001 through 2004 and a decrease in 2005 is seen in men but not in women and in people 45–49 and 50–54 years old but not at other ages. The linear trend from 2001 to 2004 was not apparent in the four individual regions.

The total observed number of cases in the 2 months of 2005 (1,488) was lower than the number expected from linear regression (1,690), and this indicates a significant 13.1% decrease in the rate (standardized incidence ratio [SIR], 0.86; 95% CI, 0.83–0.92). When the data were analyzed by sex, the decrease was statistically significant in men (SIR, 0.85; 95% CI, 0.81–0.91) but not in women (SIR, 0.98; 95% CI, 0.87–1.11). With respect to age ranges, statistically significant decreases were seen in 45- to 49-year-olds (SIR, 0.77; 95% CI, 0.68–0.89) and 50- to 54-year-olds (SIR, 0.74; 95% CI, 0.67–0.85) but not in 40- to 44-year-olds (SIR, 0.98; 95% CI, 0.82–1.19), 55- to 59-year-olds (SIR, 0.92; 95% CI, 0.84–1.02), or 60- to 64-year-olds (SIR, 0.99; 95% CI, 0.88–1.06). Statistically significant decreases from the expected rate occurred in Piedmont (SIR, 0.79; 95% CI, 0.72–0.90), Latium (SIR, 0.89; 95% CI, 0.82–0.99), and Campania (SIR, 0.89; 95% CI, 0.83–0.98) but not in Friuli–Venezia–Giulia (SIR, 0.92; 95% CI, 0.78–1.13).

Limitations of the analysis include the lack of a control population (the ban was nationwide) and the lack of information on individual smoking status. Individual exposures to secondhand smoke were also not recorded. The study also has many of the other potential limitations of an observational pre–post study based on claims information as outlined for the Helena, Montana, study.

Barone-Adesi et al. (2006) published the first report on the effect of the Italian smoking ban on acute coronary events, looking at data from the Piedmont region. The Piedmont region is one of the regions reported on by Vasselli et al. The authors used hospital admission records from the regional hospital discharge registry for Piedmont residents who had a primary discharge diagnosis code of acute MI (*International Classification of Diseases, Revision 9, Clinical Modification [ICD-9-CM]* 410) during January 2001 and June 2005 and hospital deaths due to acute MI, and they calculated age-standardized rates of admission. A total of 17,153 cases were included in the report.

The authors found that age-standardized rates of acute MI admission decreased significantly in people less than 60 years old after the smoking ban took effect (rate ratio, 0.89; 95% CI, 0.81–0.98); decreases were found in both women (rate ratio, 0.75; 95% CI, 0.58–0.96) and men (rate ratio, 0.91; 95% CI, 0.82–1.01). The data indicate that much of the overall result was driven by changes in women. In response to questions from the committee, the authors indicated (personal communication, F. Barone-Adesi, University of Turin, January 23, 2009) that an age cut point of 60 years was chosen in advance to obtain enough cases of acute MI in both age categories (under 60 years of age and 60 years of age or older) to allow analysis. In the publication, the authors hypothesize that the differences were seen because there was a "greater effect of the ban on the habits of younger persons." Other studies did not stratify results the same way, which increases the differences across studies, but many of the studies were being conducted at the same time it would not always have been possible for researchers to design their study on the basis of the other studies. They also provided additional data analyses in which the age of 70 years was used as a cut point and that showed a similar modification of the effect by age. No decrease was seen before the ban (October–December 2004 versus October–December 2003) or in people at least 60 years old; the rate ratio in older women after implementation of the ban was 1.05 (95% CI, 0.97–1.14), in older men after implementation was 1.03 (95% CI, 0.96–1.11), and in older women and men combined after implementation was 1.05 (95% CI, 1.00–1.11).

Study limitations include those previously outlined in connection with the larger Vasselli et al. (2008) study.

Cesaroni et al. (2008) analyzed data on the frequency of acute coronary events in Rome after the introduction of the Italian ban on smoking in all indoor public places. Rome is part of the Latium region of Italy that was included by Vasselli et al. (2008). The authors used two population registers—the hospital discharge database and the regional mortality register—to obtain information on the number of acute coronary events in residents of Rome in 2000–2005. All discharges that had a principal diagnosis of acute MI (*ICD-9-CM* 410) or a secondary diagnosis of acute MI when the principal diagnosis indicated acute MI complications (for example, *ICD-9-CM* 427.1 for paroxysmal ventricular tachycardia, *ICD-9-CM* 427.41 for ventricular fibrillation, *ICD-9-CM* 427.42 for ventricular flutter, and *ICD-9-CM* 427.5 for cardiac arrest) were defined as hospitalizations for acute coronary events. A total of 40,314 cases in 2000–2005 were analyzed for the publication. The period of followup after implementation of the ban was just under 12 months. Any event that occurred within 28 days of an event in the same person was not counted (was not considered to be an independent event). To try to control for confounding, the authors collected daily mean data on PM_{10} particles from four fixed monitors and data on cigarette sales in Rome and smoking habits based on health surveys provided by the National Institute of Statistics. The authors computed age-standardized annual rates of acute coronary events by using a Poisson regression analysis and adjusting for calendar time.

A statistically significant decrease in acute coronary events occurred after implementation of the smoking ban in 35- to 64-year-olds (relative risk [RR], 0.89; 95% CI, 0.85–0.93) and in 65- to 74-year-olds (RR, 0.92; 95% CI, 0.88–0.97). There was no such association in those over 74 years old. Data on smokers' deaths from coronary heart disease show RRs decreasing with age (Burns, 2003). If the oldest group and the younger groups differ in lifestyle (for example, time spent in restaurants and in bars), that could influence the effect of the ban on the different age groups. It should be noted, however, that there appeared to be a decline in heart-attack rates even before the ban. The authors conducted an analysis that was adjusted for that long-term trend, and the decrease was significant even after that adjustment. The effect was greatest in lower socioeconomic categories and was statistically significant in men but not in women; however, analysis of the interactions with socioeconomic status and sex were not statistically significant. Both smoking prevalence and cigarette sales decreased during the study period.

Cesaroni et al. (2008) assessed outcomes in a period of 12 months, longer than the 2 months of Vasselli et al. (2008) and the 6 months of Barone-Adesi et al. (2006), but did not have as broad a population base (only Rome) as the analysis of data on four Italian regions by Vasselli et al. (2008). Although there was no concurrent control population, it controlled for potential confounders that included particulate matter (only PM_{10}), an influenza epidemic, holidays, and air temperature. There was no information on individual smoking status, but the authors did use information on smoking prevalence in Rome and the RRs posed by active smoking to estimate the extent of the decrease in acute coronary events that might be attributable to smoking cessation; they estimated that less than 2% of the decrease was attributable to smoking cessation. The study included fatal and nonfatal acute MIs and a large population. The authors explained the rationale for including both primary and secondary events. Although it is good that troponin test results were used in diagnosing acute MIs, use of this method alone could result in misdiagnosing as acute MIs some events that are not acute MIs inasmuch as troponin can also be increased in some systemic diseases and in nonthrombotic cardiac disease (Inbar and Shoenfeld, 2009) and small changes can occur in clinically stable populations (Eggers et al., 2009).

PUEBLO, COLORADO

Smoking Ban and Exposure Information

The city of Pueblo, Colorado, implemented a smoking ordinance, effective July 1, 2003, that prohibited smoking in workplaces and all public buildings (including restaurants, bars, bowling alleys, and other business establishments). The committee did not identify any air or biomonitoring studies in Pueblo. The ordinance was implemented after a vote that indicated public support for the ban, and Bartecchi et al. (2006) reported that "Pueblo law enforcement officials strongly supported the ordinance and imposed significant fines on violators and on facility owners who allowed smoking on their premises."

Two publications report on acute coronary events after implementation of the smoking ban: Bartecchi et al. (2006) and Centers for Disease Control and Prevention (CDC, 2009). Both provide information directly related to the association between smoking bans and acute coronary events. The CDC study included 3 years of followup after implementation of the ban; the earlier publication reported data after 1.5 years of followup.

Published Results on Acute Coronary Events

CDC (2009) studied the effect of the citywide smoking ordinance on the incidence of acute MI–related hospitalizations in the city. The authors assessed patients who had a primary diagnosis of acute MI (*ICD-9* 410.xx) and were admitted to Parkview Medical Center or St. Mary-Corwin Medical Center in 2002–2004; cases were not confirmed clinically. Cases in three periods were assessed: the 1.5 years before implementation of the ban on July 1, 2003 (January 2002–June 2003); the 1.5 years after July 1, 2003 (July 2003–December 2004; phase I post-implementation data previously published in Bartecchi et al. [2006]; and the 1.5 years after that (January 2005–June 30, 2006; phase II post-implementation data). Information on admission date, primary diagnosis, sex, age, *ICD* code, and hospital name was collected; no information on individual smoking status was available. The authors classified patients in Pueblo County as residing either inside or outside the city limits on the basis of administrative data, including ZIP codes. To allow comparison, the authors also assessed rates of hospitalization for acute MI in a geographically isolated community, El Paso County,

Colorado. Pueblo County and El Paso County are each served by only two hospitals.

Hospitalizations for acute MI decreased from 257/100,000 person-years in the 1.5 years before implementation to 187/100,000 and 152/100,000 person-years in phase I and phase II, respectively. Those decreases represent an RR for phase I of 0.73 (95% CI, 0.64–0.82) compared with the risk before implementation and RRs in phase II of 0.81 (95% CI, 0.67–0.96) compared with phase I and 0.59 (95% CI, 0.49–0.70) compared with the period before implementation. No significant decreases were seen in Pueblo County outside the Pueblo city limits (RR ranged from 0.85 with a 95% CI of 0.56–1.14 to 1.03 with a 95% CI of 0.68–1.39) or in El Paso County (RR ranged from 0.95 with a 95% CI of 0.87–1.03 to 0.99 with a 95% CI of 0.91–1.08). The authors also obtained data on the numbers of deaths from acute MI in Pueblo from the Health Statistics Section of the Colorado Department of Public Health and Environment. Assuming that all fatal acute MIs occurred in people who did not reach the hospital and adding those numbers to the numbers of cases based on admission data, the authors reported that the phase II RR remained statistically significant both when compared with phase I (RR, 0.82; 95% CI, 0.64–0.97) and when compared with the pre-implementation period (RR, 0.66; 95% CI, 0.55–0.77).

The CDC study (CDC, 2009) adds to the information on Colorado by extending the period looked at after implementation of the smoking ban from that published by Bartecchi et al. (2006). Bartecchi et al. (2006) evaluated acute MI hospitalization rates 1.5 years before and 1.5 years after enforcement of the smoke-free ordinance. They identified a total of 2,794 patients who had a primary diagnosis of acute MI during the period of interest: 690 who resided inside the Pueblo city limits, 165 patients outside the Pueblo city limits but in Pueblo County, and 1,939 in El Paso County. There was a significant difference in sex distribution in the patients in the three locations (p = 0.003): a higher proportion of female acute MI patients (40.9%) within the Pueblo city limits than outside the city limits (33.3%) or in El Paso County (33.7%). The results were similar to those of CDC with minor differences due to record updating. Bartecchi et al. (2006) found a decrease in acute MI hospitalizations in those residing within the Pueblo city limits after enforcement of the smoke-free ordinance, from 257 before the ban to 187 after implementation (RR, 0.73; 95% CI, 0.63–0.85). A significant decrease in acute MI hospitalizations remained after adjustment for season (RR, 0.74; 95% CI, 0.64–0.86). The authors did not find a significant decrease in residents outside the city limits (from 132 to 112; RR, 0.85; 95% CI, 0.63–1.16; adjusted RR, 0.87; 95% CI, 0.64–1.17) or in El Paso County (from 119 to 116;

RR, 0.97; 95% CI, 0.89–1.06; adjusted RR, 0.99; 95% CI, 0.90–1.08). There was, however, a significant difference in the reduction in acute MI hospitalization rate between those residing within the Pueblo city limits and those in El Paso County (p < 0.001).

The two studies had the same strengths and limitations. They both had pre-implementation and postimplementation information and a concurrent control group, and the authors adjusted for out-of-hospital deaths, season, and county population. The smoking rate in El Paso County, the concurrent control group, however, increased from 17.4% (95% CI, 14.5–20.2%) to 22.3% (95% CI, 19.3–25.4%), whereas the rate in Pueblo County (including the city of Pueblo) decreased from 25.9% (95% CI, 20.2–31.6%) to 20.6% (95% CI, 15.4–25.8%) (CDC, 2009). The trends in the smoking rates could affect the estimated changes in acute MI in comparisons between the two counties. The authors note that the decrease in Pueblo County was not significant but do not comment on the change in El Paso County. Data on changes in smoking rates in Pueblo city itself, the location of the ordinance, were not available. It is unknown to what extent Pueblo County residents who do not live in Pueblo city work or spend time in Pueblo city. If a substantial number of county residents spend time in the city that could affect comparisons by biasing towards the null. The authors did not confirm the definition of acute MI by verifying an *ICD-9* code and did not provide retrospective results from Pueblo for trends in acute MI admissions. The studies lacked information on variant risk factors at the patient level, including changes in smoking status. The authors did not quantify exposure or adjust for air-pollutant concentrations, although they noted that the inclusion of a control county may have accounted for fluctuations in air quality. The studies did not account for confounders that could include prevention activities and pollution reduction in Pueblo or migration. The statistical model that accounted for season demonstrated a poor fit with only 1 degree of freedom.

MONROE COUNTY, INDIANA

Smoking Ban and Exposure Information

Monroe County, Indiana, implemented a ban on smoking in all restaurants, retail stores, and workplaces effective August 1, 2003; the ban was extended to bars on January 1, 2005. One publication examined the relationship between the smoking ban and acute coronary events (Seo and Torabi, 2007). The committee was unable to find any published information on decreased concentrations of secondhand-smoke components or compliance with the Monroe County ban.

Published Results on Acute Coronary Events

Seo and Torabi (2007) used an ex post facto matched–control-group design to assess the effect of a smoking ban on admissions of nonsmoking patients for acute MI; thus, their study directly addressed the question of the association between secondhand-smoke exposure and acute coronary events. The study population included nonsmoking patients admitted to two Monroe County hospitals—Bloomington Hospital and Ball Memorial Hospital—with a primary or secondary diagnosis of acute MI.[1] The authors assessed admission rates during two periods: period 1 consisted of 22 months before enforcement of the original smoking ban in Monroe County (August 2001–May 2003), and period 2 consisted of the 22 months after the beginning of enforcement (August 2003–May 2005). The authors selected Delaware County, Indiana, as the comparison county because it is geographically distant from Monroe County but similar to it in the percentage of the population living in urban areas, demographic profile, median household income, and mortality from heart disease and cancer.

The authors collected patient information from the hospitals, including admission date, smoking status, information on comorbidities, cardiac history, diagnosis, and laboratory values, such as troponin I and creatine phosphokinase concentrations. The criteria for patient selection included "1) a primary or secondary diagnosis of acute MI (*ICD-9-CM* codes 410.xx); 2) no past cardiac procedure that could have precipitated acute MI; 3) no comorbidity such as hypertension and high cholesterol that could have precipitated acute MI; 4) chemical evidence such as increased troponin I concentrations or creatine phosphokinase activity; and 5) onset of symptoms in the study area." The committee noted that those exclusions would eliminate detection of any effects that secondhand smoke might have on the population predisposed to an acute MI.

The authors found a significant decline (12 fewer admissions; 95% CI, 2.81–21.19) in admissions of nonsmoking patients for acute MI from period 1 (17 admissions) to period 2 (5 admissions). In contrast, there was a nonsignificant decline (2 fewer admissions; 95% CI, –13.43 to 9.43) in admissions of nonsmoking patients in Delaware County from period 1 (18 admissions) to period 2 (16 admissions). The authors found no significant difference in nonsmoking-patient admissions during period 1 between Monroe County and Delaware County. However, there was a significant

---

[1] The committee contacted a study author for more information on comorbidities. The author stated that cases with comorbidities were excluded to avoid attributing to secondhand-smoke exposure heart attacks that might have had other underlying causes. The authors excluded people who had systolic blood pressure above 140 mmHg and those with total cholesterol above 200 mg/dL (personal communication, Dr. Seo, Indiana University, Bloomington, February 9, 2009).

difference in nonsmoking-patient admissions between the counties during period 2 (5 admissions in Monroe County and 16 in Delaware County).

The study's focus on nonsmokers strengthened its relevance for answering the question of the effect of a decrease in secondhand-smoke exposure, but exclusion of cases with comorbidities could exclude cases in which secondhand smoke triggered an event in a person predisposed to an acute MI, and it greatly reduced the sample size. Smoking status was determined on the basis of admission records, so there might have been misclassification. Most studies, however, including a review and meta-analysis of 26 published studies (Patrick et al., 1994) and more recent studies (Martinez et al., 2004; Studts et al., 2006), have demonstrated minimal or low underreporting of current smoking status, although others report that underreporting of smoking is significant in England and Poland but not in the United States (Lewis et al., 2003; West et al., 2007) or is rare but possibly increasing (Fendrich et al., 2005). A longer period of followup after implementation of the smoking ban would permit a fuller assessment of its impact on acute MI–related hospital admissions. In addition, Teo and Sorabi (2007) showed unusually small numbers of acute MI events in nonsmokers (for example, no admissions for acute MI in nonsmokers in Monroe County since January 1, 2005). With respect to the analysis, the authors compare the difference in acute MIs before and after the ban in Monroe County, and compare the number of acute MIs after the ban in Monroe County to Delaware County (a county with a similar population for which there were no significant differences in acute MIs prior to the ban in Monroe County, that did not implement a smoking ban). Both of those analyses, however, can have problems. Trends over time (for example, if the rate of acute MIs was decreasing prior to the implementation of the smoking ban) could confound the first analysis; differences between the two counties could confound the second analysis. A "differences-in-differences" analysis, which tests whether the differences between the decreases in the two counties are significant, would be a preferable analysis that would control for those potential confounders. Such an analysis is often conducted on observational data in social sciences to examine the effects of a program or policy change (Buckley and Shang, 2003).

BOWLING GREEN, OHIO

Smoking Restriction and Exposure Information

The city of Bowling Green, Ohio, implemented a clean-indoor-air ordinance in March 2002 that banned smoking in all public places in the city except bars, restaurants with bars in isolated areas, and bowling alleys. Bars and bowling alleys allowed smoking at the owners' discretion.

One publication examines acute coronary events after implementation of the ordinance (Khuder et al., 2007). It provides information directly related to the question of the association between smoking bans and acute coronary events. The publication contains no information on compliance with the restrictions or on air monitoring or biomonitoring before or after the ban. Akbar-Khanzadeh et al. (2004), however, measured the concentrations of secondhand-smoke–related compounds in restaurants in Toledo and Bowling Green, Ohio, using standard methods (including nicotine, 3-ethenylpyridine, total respirable suspended particulate matter [RSP], RSP based on solanesol particles, respirable suspended ultraviolet-absorbing particulate matter, and fluorescent particulate matter). One smoke-free restaurant and one smoking restaurant (that is, with a bar) in each city were chosen. Data from a previous study were compared with data on average concentrations of the various compounds in the two cities combined. Analyses indicated that the concentrations of secondhand-smoke–related contaminants did not change after the adoption of the smoking restrictions, but the data also indicated that the concentrations of secondhand-smoke–related compounds were lower in the nonsmoking restaurants than in the restaurants that allowed smoking in separate areas.

Published Results on Acute Coronary Events

Khuder at al. (2007) compared hospital admissions related to coronary heart disease (CHD; *ICD-9-CM* 410–414, 428) in Bowling Green, Ohio, with a matched control city, Kent, Ohio, over a 6.5-year period to assess the effect of the ordinance. The study took advantage of a natural experiment. The authors obtained hospital discharge data on residents of the two cities from all hospitals in Ohio and analyzed the primary diagnoses for admission of people at least 18 years old, using 2000 census population information as the denominator throughout the study period. The authors present annual standardized admission rates in their Table 1, in which the data for the first half of 2005 are doubled to provide numbers for the full year. Despite showing those annual rates, they used monthly time-series data for the analysis in the study, and only the available data for 2005 were used. They calculated age-standardized rates and found that CHD admission rates decreased significantly in Bowling Green after the implementation and enforcement of the smoking restrictions by 39% from 2002 (36/10,000 residents) to 2003 (22/10,000 residents) and by 47% from 2002 to the first half of 2005 (19/10,000 residents). Kent did not show any significant change in CHD admission rates, nor did admission rates for causes unrelated to smoking change significantly in either city. In addition, in November 2002, 7 months after implementation of the restrictions, the monthly admission rates for CHD in Bowling Green showed a significant decline (the value of the parameter representing a change in the series level, ω, was -1.69; $p = 0.04$).

The results of the study have to be understood in relation to its limitations: the residents of Kent were assumed not to be affected by the restrictions, other risk factors for CHD may have affected admission rates, and smoking status and exposure to secondhand smoke were not accounted for. The study showed a peak in acute MIs in 2002, the year with which postimplementation years are being compared. The smoking ban was implemented in March 2002, but, on the basis of previous studies, the authors "postulated that at least 6 months would be needed to allow for the potential health effects from reduction in exposure to second hand smoke, reduction in smoking prevalence and smokers reducing the quantity of cigarettes smoked." The authors therefore "waited until October 2002 before assessing the impact of the ordinance." The sensitivity of the analysis to that choice would have been helpful to see. Annual standardized admission rates varied greatly across years, but the Autoregressive Integrated Moving Average (ARIMA) model used to analyze the data, which estimates the effect of the intervention and accounts for residual correlation, would take that variability into account. The published report provides little information on the fit of the time-series model used to measure the effect of the restrictions. As with Seo and Torabi (2007), a differences-in-differences analysis, as is often used to evaluate the effect of a program (Buckley and Shang, 2003), could have been explored, but it is not clear how it would be done with the information provided in the publication.

NEW YORK STATE

Smoking Ban and Exposure Information

On July 24, 2003, New York implemented a statewide ban on smoking in all workplaces, including restaurants, bars, and gaming establishments. Statewide smoking restrictions implemented in 1989 had limited or prohibited smoking in particular public places, such as schools, hospitals, public buildings, and retail stores. By 1995, countywide restrictions had begun to be put into place; by 2002, 75% of residents of New York state were subject to local restrictions more stringent than the statewide restrictions implemented in 1989 (Juster et al., 2007).

Juster et al. (2007) published the only report on the effect of the New York state smoking ban on acute coronary events. The authors did not measure compliance, enforcement, or markers of secondhand-smoke exposure for the report, but they cited a report by RTI International (2004) that showed that 93% of restaurants, bars, and bowling facilities were in compliance in the year after implementation. They took into consideration preexisting smoking bans, and they collected information on those bans and categorized them as comprehensive (including the statewide ban and the preexisting bans in Nassau County and New York City) or moderate[2] (all other county bans). Their report provides information directly related to questions about the association between smoking bans and acute coronary events.

Other data on compliance and potential secondhand-smoke exposure in New York state are available. The New York Adults Tobacco Survey showed decreases in saliva cotinine from 0.078 ng/mL (range, 0.054–0.111 ng/mL) to 0.041 ng/mL (0.036–0.047 ng/mL) in a sample of New York state adults before and after implementation of the ban, respectively (CDC, 2007). That study also surveyed participants about exposures to secondhand smoke. The number of respondents reporting exposure to secondhand smoke in restaurants and bars decreased significantly after implementation of the ban—in restaurants, from 19.8% reporting exposure (95% CI, 15.6–24.1%) before the ban to 3.1% (95% CI, 2.0–4.2%) 9–10 months after implementation; in bars, from 52.4% reporting exposure (95% CI, 41.5–63.4%) before the ban to 13.4% (95% CI, 9.5–17.3%) 9–10 months after implementation. However, those reporting exposure in the workplace did not decrease significantly[3]—from 13.6% reporting exposure before the ban (95% CI, 8.1–19.1%) to 7.6% (95% CI, 5.1–10.2%) 9–10 months after implementation.

CDC (2004) measured indoor-air quality in hospitality venues in western New York before and after implementation of the 2003 ban. Average $PM_{2.5}$ concentration decreased from 324 $\mu g/m^3$ before the ban to 25 $\mu g/m^3$ after implementation (p < 0.001).

Published Results on Acute Coronary Events

Juster et al. (2007) assessed the effect of the statewide smoking ban in New York on hospital admissions for acute MI and stroke. The authors analyzed monthly hospital admissions associated with primary diagnoses of acute MI (ICD-9-CM 410.0–410.99) and stroke (ICD-9-CM 430.00–438.99) from January 1995 to December 2004 in 62 counties in New York state. They used data from a comprehensive database maintained by the New York State Department of Health and included data from all public and private hospitals in the state. The number of hospital admissions was combined with county population data to obtain a monthly rate of hospital admissions for acute MI and stroke; the data were age-adjusted to the 2000

---

[2] The authors of the report defined a moderate ban as one that restricts smoking but provides little or no protection in hospitality venues.

[3] Statistical analysis used a t test for trend.

New York population. Multiple linear-regression analysis was applied to monthly age-adjusted county rates for acute MI and stroke, and estimated regression coefficients were used to predict the potential reduction in hospital admissions related to comprehensive and moderate smoking bans.

During the study period, there were more than 46,000 hospital admissions per year for acute MI and more than 58,000 for stroke. Regression analysis indicated that no sudden decrease in hospital admissions for acute MI was associated with the implementation of the smoking ban in 2003. However, the interaction between the law and time—assessed by comparing the changes in the slope of the line for observed versus expected events after the ban—indicated that the decline in monthly acute MIs associated with the countywide and statewide bans was greater than the decline expected in the absence of those bans. Moderate smoking bans reduced the monthly trend rate by an estimated average of 0.15/100,000 persons per month; the statewide comprehensive ban reduced the monthly trend rate by an estimated average of 0.32/100,000 per month. The analysis indicated that there were 8% (3,813) fewer hospital admissions for acute MI in 2004 in the presence of the comprehensive statewide ban than would have been expected that year with only the previous local smoking restrictions and bans in place. Although it was not reported in Juster et al. (2007), the authors stated in response to questions from this committee that a similar analysis of mortality in 1998–2005 in New York state had similar results, although an interaction between law and time did not reach significance, with a p-value of 0.059 (personal communication, H. Juster, New York State Department of Health, Albany, January 14, 2009).

At the time of the study, some partial or full bans were in place in various locations in the state before the statewide ban (that is, there was not a "zero to all" implementation throughout the state) and would be expected to affect the magnitude of any change seen. Juster et al. (2007) estimated that if no local bans had been in place when the state ban was implemented, the effect of the state ban would have been a 19% decrease in acute MIs.

The study included some measures of exposure but did not assess individual patient-level data (including smoking status or other risk factors) or the effect of changes in smoking prevalence on hospital admissions. There was no control for repeat admissions of the same person. The considerable data aggregation in the study could mask heterogeneity and overstate statistical significance. From the data in Figure 1 of Juster et al. (2007), it appears that the effect of the ban on acute MIs and stroke was not immediate: an apparently anomalous initial drop in both observed admissions and admissions expected in the absence of the statewide ban (as predicted by the model) was followed by a separation between the observed occurrences with the statewide ban and the expected number in the absence of the ban. The committee notes, however, that whereas typically the rate of acute

MI is much greater than (as much as twice as high as) the rate of strokes (Lloyd-Jones et al., 2008), in this study there were more strokes than acute MIs. With respect to the analyses, this was the only study that attempted to account for previously implemented smoking bans; that is important given the large portion of the study population that was previously covered by smoking bans (New York City and several other large jurisdictions had previously implemented smoking bans). The results of the study, however, are sensitive to the assumptions used in the model and to the model choice. A sensitivity analysis showing the effect of model choice on study results might have provided more confidence in the study findings.

SASKATCHEWAN, CANADA

Smoking Ban and Exposure Information

Saskatoon, Saskatchewan, Canada, implemented a smoking ban on July 1, 2004. The ban prohibited smoking in "any enclosed public space that is open to the public or to which the public is customarily admitted or invited." Smoking was also prohibited in outdoor seating areas of restaurants and licensed premises. Smoking had previously been prohibited in government buildings.

Lemstra et al. (2008) conducted the only study to assess whether the smoking ban had an effect on rates of acute MI and also assessed smoking prevalence and public support of the ban. That study provides information directly related to questions about the association between smoking bans and acute coronary events. The authors measured business compliance with the ban by reviewing warnings and tickets issued by public-health inspectors to eligible businesses. Of 924 eligible establishments, 914 (98.9%) were inspected within the first 6 months of the ban. Of the 914, only 13 (1.4%) had to be issued noncompliance warnings (for not posting signs or removing ashtrays); one ticket was issued on reinspection of those 13 that were issued warnings. The committee found no exposure-assessment data.

Published Results on Acute Coronary Events

Lemstra et al. (2008) obtained information on acute MI from the Strategic Health Information Planning Services. *ICD-10* codes, rather than *ICD-9* codes, were in use in Saskatoon beginning in 2000, so the analyses used data from July 2000 and later. The authors calculated age-standardized incidences of acute MI per 100,000 people in the first full year of the smoking ban (July 1, 2004–June 30, 2005) and in the previous 4 years (July 1, 2000–June 30, 2004). Data collected on smoking prevalence in 2003 and 2005 by Statistics Canada were used to evaluate changes in smoking pattern.

The age-standardized incidence of acute MI decreased from 176.1 cases/100,000 people before the ban to 152.4 cases/100,000 after implementation of the ban. The 13% reduction was statistically significant (rate ratio, 0.87; 95% CI, 0.84–0.90). Smoking prevalence in Saskatoon decreased from 24.1% in 2003 to 18.2% in 2005 but was unchanged in the province of Saskatchewan.

The study contained some information available from a survey that determined changes in active smoking status (for example, a decrease in the number of people who actively smoked and a decrease in the number of cigarettes smoked by the people who continued to smoke). In addition, the study had a large sample and comprehensive data. The study accounted for changes in *ICD* coding for acute MI, choosing its timeframe on the basis, in part, of the coding change. The study has a number of limitations: no information on individual exposure to secondhand smoke was available, the postimplementation study period was brief, and no comparison city was available to permit assessment of trends or of any long-term decline.

SCOTLAND

Smoking Ban and Exposure Information

Scotland prohibited smoking in enclosed public places and workplaces— including bars, restaurants, and cafes—as of March 2006. As described by Haw and Gruer (2007), the exceptions included "residential accommodation and designated rooms in hotels, care homes, hospices, and psychiatric units." Pell et al. (2008) conducted the only study that assessed the effects of that ban on acute coronary events. The study surveyed participants on smoking status and secondhand-smoke exposure before and after the ban, and it measured serum cotinine. The correlation between self-reported duration of exposure to secondhand smoke and serum cotinine concentrations was similar before ($r = 0.33$, $p < 0.001$) and after ($r = 0.33$, $p < 0.001$) the implementation of the smoking ban. The number of never-smokers who reported no exposure to smoke increased from 57% before the ban to 78% after implementation ($p < 0.001$) largely because of reduced exposure to smoke in pubs, bars, and clubs. The geometric mean of individual serum cotinine measurements in never-smokers decreased from 0.68 to 0.56 ng/mL ($p < 0.001$) after implementation. Participants identified as former smokers showed similar changes before and after implementation. Those data indicate that secondhand-smoke exposure decreased in the study population after implementation.

Other published research supports the conclusion that secondhand-smoke exposure decreased in Scotland after implementation of the ban. Semple et al. (2007a) monitored $PM_{2.5}$ during 53 visits to 41 pubs in

Edinburgh and Aberdeen both before implementation of the ban and 2 months after implementation; particulate matter is one component of secondhand smoke. Air samples were collected for a minimum of 30 min; days of the week and times of day of sampling before and after implementation were matched. Before the ban, $PM_{2.5}$ concentrations were 8–902 $\mu g/m^3$; after implementation, they were 6–104 $\mu g/m^3$. With the exception of one bar that had a very low $PM_{2.5}$ concentration before the ban and only a slightly lower concentration after implementation, $PM_{2.5}$ concentrations decreased by at least 50% in all establishments; in more than half, concentrations decreased by at least 90%. The researchers also collected information on compliance with the ban while conducting the sampling. Only 1 of the 41 pubs had evidence of smoking after implementation of the ban.

Haw and Gruer (2007) measured changes in exposure to secondhand smoke in the 14 regions of Scotland. Using a repeat, cross-sectional design, the researchers interviewed adults (ages 16–74 years) on health behaviors, smoking status, nicotine-replacement therapy use, and reported exposures to secondhand smoke before and after implementation of the ban. They also measured cotinine concentrations in saliva samples. Nonsmokers reported decreased exposure to secondhand smoke after implementation of the ban. When sex, years of education, and deprivation of residence (subjects were categorized according to how affluent or deprived their residences were) were controlled for, self-reported decreases were significant only for public places covered by the ban (including pubs, work, and public transport) and not in private homes and cars. In nonsmokers, the geometric mean cotinine concentration decreased by 39% (p < 0.001), from 0.43 ng/mL before the ban to 0.26 ng/mL after implementation. Nonsmokers not living with any smokers showed a greater reduction than nonsmokers living with at least one smoker, with a 49% reduction (95% CI, 40–56%; p < 0.001) and a 16% reduction (95% CI, –11 to 37%; p < 0.05), respectively.

Menzies et al. (2006) measured serum cotinine concentrations in bar workers in Dundee and Perth, Scotland, and found that concentrations decreased by 1.93 ng/mL (95% CI, 1.03–2.83 ng/mL; p < 0.001), from 5.15 ng/mL before the ban to 3.22 ng/mL 1 month after implementation, and by 2.22 ng/mL (95% CI, 1.34–3.10 ng/mL; p < 0.001), to 2.93 ng/mL 2 months after implementation. They also found that respiratory symptoms had decreased and pulmonary function improved at both 1 and 2 months after implementation relative to 1 month before implementation.

Semple et al. (2007b) met with 371 people who worked in 72 bars in Aberdeen, Glasgow, Edinburgh, and small towns in two rural areas of Scotland before implementation of the ban (January–March 2006) and twice after implementation (May–July 2006 and January–March 2007). Salivary cotinine in 301 workers was assayed. The geometric mean salivary cotinine concentration in nonsmokers decreased from 2.9 ng/mL before the ban to

0.7 ng/mL about 2 months after implementation to 0.4 ng/mL about a year after implementation.

Pell et al. (2008) measured serum cotinine concentrations in the study that evaluated acute MI. The concentration of cotinine in serum samples validated self-reported smoking status and provided a measure of exposure to secondhand smoke; serum cotinine decreased by 38% in men and by 47% in women after implementation of the ban. For the purposes of the study, current smokers were those who reported being smokers and had serum cotinine greater than 12 ng/mL. Never-smokers reported never having smoked and had serum cotinine of no more than 12 ng/mL. Former smokers reported being former smokers and had serum cotinine of no more than 12 ng/mL.

Published Results on Acute Coronary Events

Pell et al. (2008) prospectively examined the number of hospital admissions for acute coronary syndrome before and after implementation of smoking ban. Their study had serum cotinine concentrations of patients and analyzed the data according to smoking status on the basis of those concentrations, so it directly addressed the question of the association between secondhand-smoke exposure and acute coronary events. The authors gathered information on cases from nine hospitals during the 10 months before implementation (June 2005–March 2006) and 10 months after (June 2006–March 2007). They used detection of cardiac troponin after emergency admission for chest pain to define an acute coronary syndrome; cardiac troponin is routinely measured in people who are admitted with chest pain. During the pre-implementation and postimplementation periods, there were 3,235 and 2,684 admissions for acute coronary syndrome, respectively, in the nine hospitals (the nine hospitals accounted for 64% of admissions for acute coronary syndrome in Scotland). Pell et al. (2008) used English hospitals' admissions for acute coronary syndrome as a concurrent control.

The number of admissions for acute coronary syndrome decreased by 17% (95% CI, 16–18%). Only a 4% reduction occurred during the same period in England, where no ban was in place. In the 10 years before implementation of the ban, a trend of a 3% mean reduction per year occurred in Scotland. Examination by smoking status showed a 14% reduction in smokers, 19% in former smokers, and 21% in those who never smoked; the data indicate that 67% of the prevented admissions were in nonsmokers.

This study was one of the few that used a prospective design to address the question of the effect of a smoking ban on acute coronary events. It has several strengths, including a large sample, laboratory confirmation of MI admissions with cardiac troponin assays, and confirmation that there was no concurrent change in the rates of out-of-hospital deaths after implementation of the ban. The authors also conducted a survey of cases and a sample of the general population for secondhand-smoke exposure and smoking status, and they measured cotinine concentrations in these participants.

The study did, however, have limitations. Although it was large, it did not include all hospitals in Scotland, it did not have a clearly defined study population, and there could have been changes in the nine hospital catchment areas or a more general population influx or efflux after implementation of the ban. The study had a relatively short followup period (1 year), so the long-term effect of the ban on smokers and nonsmokers is not known. It is unclear whether the ban itself affected smoking status in the general population by changing social norms. Finally, as in all observational trials, other changes—including changes in health-care availability and in the standard of practice in cardiac care, such as new diagnostic criteria for acute MI—during the study period could have confounded the results.

REFERENCES

Akbar-Khanzadeh, F., S. Milz, A. Ames, S. Spino, and C. Tex. 2004. Effectiveness of clean indoor air ordinances in controlling environmental tobacco smoke in restaurants. *Archives of Environmental Health* 59(12):677-685.

ANRF (American Nonsmokers' Rights Foundation). 2009. *Chronological table of U.S. population protected by 100% smokefree state or local laws.* (Accessed July 2, 2009, from http://www.no-smoke.org/goingsmokefree.php?id=519.)

Barone-Adesi, F., L. Vizzini, F. Merletti, and L. Richiardi. 2006. Short-term effects of Italian smoking regulation on rates of hospital admission for acute myocardial infarction. *European Heart Journal* 27(20):2468-2472.

Bartecchi, C., R. N. Alsever, C. Nevin-Woods, W. M. Thomas, R. O. Estacio, B. B. Bartelson, and M. J. Krantz. 2006. Reduction in the incidence of acute myocardial infarction associated with a citywide smoking ordinance. *Circulation* 114(14):1490-1496.

Buckley, J., and Y. Shang. 2003. Estimating policy and program effects with observational data: The "Differences-in-differences" Estimator. *Practical Assessment, Research & Evaluation* 8(24). (Accessed May 21, 2009, from http://PAREonline.net/getvn.asp?v=8&n=24.)

Burns, D. M. 2003. Epidemiology of smoking-induced cardiovascular disease. *Progress in Cardiovascular Diseases* 46(1):11-29.

CDC (Centers for Disease Control and Prevention). 2004. Indoor air quality in hospitality venues before and after implementation of a clean indoor air law—western New York, 2003. *MMWR—Morbidity & Mortality Weekly Report* 53(44):1038-1041.

———. 2007. Reduced secondhand smoke exposure after implementation of a comprehensive statewide smoking ban—New York, June 26, 2003–June 30, 2004. *MMWR—Morbidity & Mortality Weekly Report* 56(28):705-708.

———. 2009. Reduced hospitalizations for acute myocardial infarction after implementation of a smoke-free ordinance— city of Pueblo, Colorado, 2002–2006. *MMWR—Morbidity & Mortality Weekly Report* 57(51):1373-1377.

Cesaroni, G., F. Forastiere, N. Agabiti, P. Valente, P. Zuccaro, and C. A. Perucci. 2008. Effect of the Italian smoking ban on population rates of acute coronary events. *Circulation* 117(9):1183-1188.

Eggers, K. M., L. Lind, P. Venge, and B. Lindahl. 2009. Will the universal definition of myocardial infarction criteria result in an overdiagnosis of myocardial infarction? *American Journal of Cardiology* 103(5):588-591.

Fendrich, M., M. E. Mackesy-Amiti, T. P. Johnson, A. Hubbell, and J. S. Wislar. 2005. Tobacco-reporting validity in an epidemiological drug-use survey. *Addictive Behaviors* 30(1):175-181.

Gallus, S., P. Zuccaro, P. Colombo, G. Apolone, R. Pacifici, S. Garattini, and C. La Vecchia. 2006. Effects of new smoking regulations in Italy. *Annals of Oncology* 17(2):346-347.

Gorini, G., A. Gasparrini, M. C. Fondelli, A. S. Costantini, F. Centrich, M. J. Lopez, M. Nebot, and E. Tamang. 2005. Environmental tobacco smoke (ETS) exposure in Florence hospitality venues before and after the smoking ban in Italy. *Journal of Occupational & Environmental Medicine* 47(12):1207-1210.

Haw, S. J., and L. Gruer. 2007. Changes in exposure of adult non-smokers to secondhand smoke after implementation of smoke-free legislation in Scotland: National cross sectional survey. *BMJ* 335(7619):549.

Inbar, R., and Y. Shoenfeld. 2009. Elevated cardiac troponins: The ultimate marker for myocardial necrosis, but not without a differential diagnosis. *Israel Medical Association Journal: Imaj* 11(1):50-53.

Juster, H. R., B. R. Loomis, T. M. Hinman, M. C. Farrelly, A. Hyland, U. E. Bauer, and G. S. Birkhead. 2007. Declines in hospital admissions for acute myocardial infarction in New York state after implementation of a comprehensive smoking ban. *American Journal of Public Health* 97(11):2035-2039.

Khuder, S. A., S. Milz, T. Jordan, J. Price, K. Silvestri, and P. Butler. 2007. The impact of a smoking ban on hospital admissions for coronary heart disease. *Preventive Medicine* 45(1):3-8.

Lemstra, M., C. Neudorf, and J. Opondo. 2008. Implications of a public smoking ban. *Canadian Journal of Public Health* 99(1):62-65.

Lewis, S. J., N. M. Cherry, R. McL Niven, P. V. Barber, K. Wilde, and A. C. Povey. 2003. Cotinine levels and self-reported smoking status in patients attending a bronchoscopy clinic. *Biomarkers* 8(3-4):218-228.

Lloyd-Jones, D., R. Adams, M. Carnethon, G. De Simone, T. B. Ferguson, K. Flegal, E. Ford, K. Furie, A. Go, K. Greenlund, N. Haase, S. Hailpern, M. Ho, V. Howard, B. Kissela, S. Kittner, D. Lackland, L. Lisabeth, A. Marelli, M. McDermott, J. Meigs, D. Mozaffarian, G. Nichol, C. O'Donnell, V. Roger, W. Rosamond, R. Sacco, P. Sorlie, R. Stafford, J. Steinberger, T. Thom, S. Wasserthiel-Smoller, N. Wong, J. Wylie-Rosett, and Y. Hong. 2008. Heart disease and stroke statistics—2009 update. A report from the American Heart Association statistics committee and stroke statistics subcommittee. *Circulation* 119:e21-e181.

Martinez, M. E., M. Reid, R. Jiang, J. Einspahr, and D. S. Alberts. 2004. Accuracy of self-reported smoking status among participants in a chemoprevention trial. *Preventive Medicine* 38(4):492-497.

Menzies, D., A. Nair, P. A. Williamson, S. Schembri, M. Z. H. Al-Khairalla, M. Barnes, T. C. Fardon, L. McFarlane, G. J. Magee, and B. J. Lipworth. 2006. Respiratory symptoms, pulmonary function, and markers of inflammation among bar workers before and after a legislative ban on smoking in public places. *JAMA* 296(14):1742-1748.

Patrick, D. L., A. Cheadle, D. C. Thompson, P. Diehr, T. Koepsell, and S. Kinne. 1994. The validity of self-reported smoking: A review and meta-analysis. *American Journal of Public Health* 84(7):1086-1093.

Pell, J. P., S. Haw, S. Cobbe, D. E. Newby, A. C. H. Pell, C. Fischbacher, A. McConnachie, S. Pringle, D. Murdoch, F. Dunn, K. Oldroyd, P. Macintyre, B. O'Rourke, and W. Borland. 2008. Smoke-free legislation and hospitalizations for acute coronary syndrome. *New England Journal of Medicine* 359(5):482-491.

RTI (Research Triangle Institute) International. 2004. *First annual independent evaluation of New York's Tobacco Control Program: Final report*. Research Triangle Park, NC.

Sargent, R. P., R. M. Shepard, and S. A. Glantz. 2004. Reduced incidence of admissions for myocardial infarction associated with public smoking ban: Before and after study. *BMJ* 328(7446):977-980.

Semple, S., K. S. Creely, A. Naji, B. G. Miller, and J. G. Ayres. 2007a. Secondhand smoke levels in Scottish pubs: The effect of smoke-free legislation. *Tobacco Control* 16(2):127-132.

Semple, S., L. Maccalman, A. A. Naji, S. Dempsey, S. Hilton, B. G. Miller, and J. G. Ayres. 2007b. Bar workers' exposure to second-hand smoke: The effect of Scottish smoke-free legislation on occupational exposure. *Annals of Occupational Hygiene* 51(7):571-580.

Seo, D.-C., and M. R. Torabi. 2007. Reduced admissions for acute myocardial infarction associated with a public smoking ban: Matched controlled study. *Journal of Drug Education* 37(3):217-226.

Studts, J. L., S. R. Ghate, J. L. Gill, C. R. Studts, C. N. Barnes, A. S. LaJoie, M. A. Andrykowski, and R. V. LaRocca. 2006. Validity of self-reported smoking status among participants in a lung cancer screening trial. *Cancer Epidemiology, Biomarkers & Prevention* 15(10):1825-1828.

Valente, P., F. Forastiere, A. Bacosi, G. Cattani, S. Di Carlo, M. Ferri, I. Figa-Talamanca, A. Marconi, L. Paoletti, C. Perucci, and P. Zuccaro. 2007. Exposure to fine and ultrafine particles from secondhand smoke in public places before and after the smoking ban, Italy 2005. *Tobacco Control* 16(5):312-317.

Vasselli, S., P. Papini, D. Gaelone, L. Spizzichino, E. De Campora, R. Gnavi, C. Saitto, N. Binkin, and G. Laurendi. 2008. Reduction incidence of myocardial infarction associated with a national legislative ban on smoking. *Minerva Cardioangiologica* 56(2):197-203.

West, R., W. Zatonski, K. Przewozniak, and M. J. Jarvis. 2007. Can we trust national smoking prevalence figures? Discrepancies between biochemically assessed and self-reported smoking rates in three countries. *Cancer Epidemiology, Biomarkers & Prevention* 16(4):820-822.

7

Synthesis of Key Studies Examining the Effect of Smoking Bans on Acute Coronary Events

In this chapter, the committee synthesizes the information yielded by the key studies and discusses the overall weight of evidence from them, their uncertainties, the extent to which the uncertainties affect interpretation of their results, and the conclusions that can be drawn from them.

LIMITATIONS AND SOURCES OF UNCERTAINTY IN KEY STUDIES

Some elements of design and uncertainty in the key studies pose challenges in the interpretation of the studies that are relevant to the effect of smoking bans on acute coronary events: the inherently nonexperimental design of the studies, the hypotheses tested in the studies, the lack of closed study populations, the use of less-than-perfect comparison groups, the need to disentangle the effects of a smoking ban itself from concurrent activities that could affect smoking behavior, exposure assessment, outcome, the time from cessation of exposure to secondhand smoke to changes in disease rates, the biologic plausibility of an effect, analytic issues, and the potential for publication bias. Those are all discussed in this section. When reviewing the key studies, the committee kept in mind the characteristics that would make an ideal study to evaluate the effect of an intervention, a smoking ban, on an outcome, acute coronary events. This was a useful framework but a caveat is needed. The committee looked at the study designs and analyses with the advantage of hindsight; such hindsight is helpful in considering how to design a more rigorous evaluation but does not imply that the study authors should have or could have designed an observational study that addressed all of those elements nor that all of those elements would have been under the control of the researchers. Those characteristics are summarized in Table 7-1. The table includes a description of the characteristics of studies and some of the ideals and challenges related to them. Researchers must weigh the benefits of those ideals across all the characteristics because a study that meets all the ideals typically will not be feasible to conduct. For example, it would be difficult to conduct a study with a large sample that requires autopsies for all cases. Furthermore, journals often have page limitations that preclude the publication of detailed analyses, such as sensitivity analyses, which ideally would be included in studies like those discussed here.

Although the 11 studies discussed here are observational studies and have limitations inherent to observational studies, it is important that the studies took advantage of natural experiments to directly evaluate the effects of an intervention (a smoking ban and concomitant activities) on a health outcome of interest (acute coronary events). As discussed in *Assessing the Health Impact of Air Quality Regulations: Concepts and Methods*

TABLE 7-1 Characteristics and Challenges in Study Design[a]

Characteristics	Ideal	Research Challenges to Consider
Study population	• Stable population • Active surveillance • Large sample • Adequate baseline data on secondhand-smoke exposure • Individual-level data (such as, smoking status, secondhand-smoke exposure, preexisting risk factors)	When using "natural" intervention, such as smoking ban, it is difficult to control many aspects of population • Population cannot be held constant, because of immigration and emigration • Active surveillance is sometimes possible but would increase costs • Sample size is limited by population covered by smoking ban • If prospective, an observational study can have baseline and individual-level data on secondhand-smoke exposure and risk factors, but is much more expensive to conduct and requires more complex human-subjects use approval • Hospital records are not always a reliable source of data on smoking status

TABLE 7-1 Continued

Characteristics	Ideal	Research Challenges to Consider
Smoking-ban intervention	• Occurs at clearly defined time • No other activities occur at same time that could affect smoking rates or secondhand-smoke exposure	• Investigators have no control over terms or timing of smoking-ban legislation, implementation, or enforcement

Exposure assessment	• Need for exposure assessment depends on hypothesis tested
	  • Exposure data not needed to test effect of smoking ban
	  • Exposure data needed to test effect of secondhand-smoke exposure
		• If study is prospective, study design can include air monitoring or biomonitoring before and after implementation of smoking ban, but increases costs and biomonitoring requires more complex human-subjects approval

Outcome	• Both morbidity and mortality data analyzed
	• Confirmation of acute coronary event:
	  • Mortality data confirmed by autopsy or independent review of medical records
	  • Acute MI data independently confirmed clinically with standardized criteria
		• Access to data is sometimes inadequate
		• It is often not practical to have autopsies conducted on all cases unless sample is very small
		• Conducting an independent review of mortality data or clinically confirming morbidity data with standardized criteria is possible but would increase costs and require more complex human-subjects approval
		• In absence of independent review, data are only as good as what is recorded

Time between implementation and effect	• Time between implementation and effect is clear	• Period between implementation and effect is difficult to establish because intervention does not occur at clearly defined time (because of other activities concurrent with ban); effect may increase over time because, for example, there are gradual changes in smoking behavior

Continued

TABLE 7-1 Continued

Characteristics	Ideal	Research Challenges to Consider
Comparison group	• Both comparison population (external control) and same population before and after implementation of intervention are used	• Use of external control population depends on availability of comparable population
Biologic plausibility	• Effect being tested is biologically plausible	• Identifying research designs that can address biologic plausibility • In hypothesis-generating studies, biologic plausibility is not always known before study is designed
Experimental design	• Experimental designs are typically best able to demonstrate cause–effect relationship	• It would not be possible ethically to test effect of secondhand smoke on acute MIs experimentally
Hypothesis clarification	• Hypothesis being tested is clearly stated • Tested hypothesis matches question being asked in interpreting results	• Studies are designed to test specific hypothesis; users of study results should consider study hypothesis when determining what questions study can answer
Statistical Design	• Appropriate statistical analysis, determined a priori, controls for appropriate confounders • Statistical models can be used to control for potential confounders and trends • Statistical modeling includes description of modeling assumptions and sensitivity analysis of impact of model choice and assumptions on modeling results	• Statistical analysis is generally under control of researchers designing study, but options could be limited by characteristics of available data • If appropriate data are available, choice of model and assumptions are under control of researchers
Publication bias	• Negative results are less apt to be published than positive findings	• Both researchers and journal editors should overcome their preference for publishing positive findings

[a] A study typically cannot attain the ideal for all characteristics, so researchers must weigh the importance of each characteristic and the availability of data when determining study design.

for Accountability Research (HEI Accountability Working Group, 2003) in the context of air-pollution regulations, studies of interventions constitute a definitive approach to determining whether regulations have health benefits. French and Heagerty (2008) also discuss the advantages and limitations of longitudinal data for assessing the impact of policy changes.

Nonexperimental Design

The key studies discussed in this report are of necessity nonexperimental; they are observational or surveillance studies that looked at the effects of a smoking ban on hospital outcomes. Such studies do not typically have a great deal of information on the individual level, including exposures and in some instances smoking status. The results of ecologic smoking-ban studies can, however, support identification of associations and findings of causality (Rubin, 2008).

Hypothesis

The majority of the key studies reviewed in this chapter were natural experiments in that there was an intervention (a smoking ban) that would lead to a reduction in secondhand-smoke exposure (with either direct evidence from a given ban or indirect evidence from bans in other locales that exposure decreased). The studies took advantage of the intervention to test the hypothesis that a reduction in secondhand-smoke exposure leads to a reduced incidence of acute coronary events. Because of a lack of information on smoking status, most of the studies did not directly address the question of whether a decrease in secondhand smoke decreases the risk of coronary events, but as discussed above, the data do indicate that secondhand-smoke exposure decreased after implementation of the bans studied; therefore, even the studies that did not have information on smoking status provide supportive evidence of the effects of secondhand smoke.

As discussed previously, only two studies (Pell et al., 2008; Seo and Torabi, 2007) had information on the smoking status of cases; therefore, only those two directly addressed the question of the effect of secondhand-smoke exposure on nonsmokers rather than the question of the effect of a smoking ban. In both of these studies a decrease in coronary events was observed among nonsmokers after implementation of the smoking ban.

It is important to consider the hypothesis tested in a study when interpreting a study. A number of different hypotheses related to secondhand-smoke exposure could be tested in a study; each would be best evaluated with a different study design, and each would be related to different questions that were asked of this committee. A cohort study could test the hypothesis that long-term exposure to secondhand smoke increases the risk of coronary events. A natural experiment (or quasiexperimental design) could be used to test the hypothesis that a long-term reduction in secondhand-smoke exposure leads to a reduced incidence of events, and a case-crossover design with a detailed examination of the temporal relationships between exposure and incidence of events would be ideal to test the hypothesis that secondhand-smoke exposure triggers acute coronary events in at-risk people (personal communication, J. Kaufman, University of Seattle, Washington, January 30, 2009). Each type of study would answer different questions that are in the charge to this committee.

Study Populations

The key studies reviewed by the committee look at different populations, or portions of populations, have different information available, and have different sample sizes, some of which are small. The differences in the populations limit the ability to quantitatively compare the changes in risk across the studies and, in some cases, limit the confidence in those studies. The studies, however, are retrospective in nature (with the exception of Scotland) and the populations are designated on the basis of the smoking ban coverage and availability of data.

The population should be large enough to minimize problems of non-uniformity over short periods, and the baseline exposure to secondhand smoke should be large enough for the study to have the power to detect changes of public-health relevance. In addition, information on the population, such as smoking status and other risk factors for acute coronary events or cardiovascular disease that could be confounders in the study, should be available.

Ideally, the study population will have been under active surveillance or enrolled in a prospective cohort study, so that the data collected before and after implementation of the ban will be directly comparable; and the population will be closed, that is, it will not change over the period of study. Inevitably, the studies that examined the effect of smoking bans were not closed populations; people were free to immigrate to or emigrate from the region studied and to move back and forth between areas with and without bans. The extent of migration in the communities studied most likely varied from study to study. However, as mentioned in Chapter 1, migration would be expected to decrease the effects of smoking bans on acute coronary events in studies unless smokers were selectively moving out of areas with bans and into areas without bans. Although none of the studies discussed the potential for migration extensively, there is no reason to believe that most of the locations would have a large amount of migration of smokers at the time of the ban and over the relatively short period of observation. One exception might be some geographic areas in New York state that are next to other states. For example, smokers in the New York City area might have lived, worked, or socialized in New Jersey (where a comprehensive statewide smoking ban was not put into effect until April 15, 2006) so that they could smoke. Other areas of the state that are farther from state borders (that is, farther from states that might not have had a smoking ban), however, have been much less likely to be affected by such migration. Similarly, people in locations that are more isolated (such as Helena, Montana, or Pueblo, Colorado) or in which bans are widely implemented (such as the entire country of Italy or Scotland) are less likely to have moved because of smoking bans. Thus, although migration in the populations studied is possible, the committee does not believe that migration biased the results of the studies substantially.

Comparison Groups

The key studies used two types of controls. Some compared acute cardiovascular events in a given population before and during smoking bans (internal control group). Such a study cannot evaluate the effects of other changes over time, and this is a concern especially because in many of the areas under study both rates of smoking and rates of acute cardiovascular disease were going down. There was an exception; one study was able to assess what happened when a ban was lifted.

Other studies, instead or in addition, selected a comparison or control population (external control group) from an area that did not implement a ban, but otherwise was similar to the population where the intervention occurred. Such a study can to some extent control for larger trends (secular trends), but the comparison populations could differ from study populations in several ways that might be relevant to the risk of exposure to secondhand smoke and to the incidence of acute cardiovascular events. This would be observed in the pre-ban comparison and would add uncertainty to the results.

A before–after comparison is useful if data on individuals are collected. If, instead, grouped population data are used in a before–after comparison, one would need to be assured that there is little mobility. Moreover, if there are other communitywide changes related to tobacco, such as a concurrent antitobacco advertising campaign, a before–after design will be less able to assess the effect of the ban independently of the other changes; a comparison with an external comparison group (not subject to a ban) may be of value so that concurrent changes can be accounted for. However, the fact that multiple studies that used internal or external control groups have found associations between smoking bans and a decrease in acute MI provides stronger evidence that the association is real and not an artifact related to the control population used.

Smoking Bans

In the 11 key reports reviewed by the committee, the effects of the interventions and the effects of events that occurred concurrently with them cannot be separately identified. Some of the studies attempted to quantify or catalog other activities that took place at the time of a smoking ban, but because the relative effects of the different activities on smoking behavior and exposures are unknown and because the activities were not independent, the committee could not attribute changes in the incidence of acute myocardial infarction (MI) to a particular aspect of a ban. The committee's conclusions are therefore based on whatever changes occurred at the time of the smoking bans and not on legislation itself.

The bans themselves were of varied scope (for example, they covered different types of sites or venues), enforcement of bans has varied, and other interventions often occurred concurrently, such as smoking-cessation and education efforts. As can be seen in Table 6-1, however, most of the bans covered workplaces, including private offices, restaurants, and bars. That could have an effect on the changes in secondhand-smoke exposure in that people could spend about 8 hours or more each day at work compared with typically many fewer hours in restaurants or bars.

In the studies reviewed in Chapter 6 there is an attempt to define clearly the specific time at which an intervention occurred. As discussed in Chapter 5, however, smoking bans typically do not occur in a vacuum, so the results of the studies need to be interpreted in the context of all activities that occurred before, after, and at the time of a legislated ban—such as public debate on the law, educational campaigns, voluntary bans in households, and increased support for smoking cessation—and not just in terms of the regulation that was implemented. For example, voluntary bans or other smoking restrictions might precede a legislated ban. The fact that other activities occurred at the same time need not weaken a study, but it can limit the conclusions that can be drawn with respect to what caused observed effects. That is, decreases in adverse health effects that occur with the implementation of a ban cannot necessarily be attributed to the specific legislation; other activities, such as voluntary bans in households or outreach programs, could underlie the effects.

Exposure Assessment

To address its charge, the committee must consider the effects of smoking bans and the effects of decreases in secondhand-smoke exposure. To do that, the committee assessed the studies to determine whether changes related to the bans are a result of changes in secondhand-smoke exposure. Ideally, in assessing the impact of a change in exposure to secondhand smoke, the size of the change in exposure would be measured to determine whether there is a dose–response relationship. Most of the key intervention studies raise two issues with regard to exposure assessment: a lack of information on the smoking status of the people with reported cases of acute MI and a lack of information on changes in secondhand-smoke exposure.

After a smoking ban is implemented, many smokers quit or decrease the number of cigarettes they smoke, and in the absence of data on smoking status it is difficult to separate a decrease in the number of cases of acute MI due to decreased exposure of nonsmokers to secondhand smoke from a decrease in the number of cases of acute MI due to decreased smoking by smokers. Two of the publications have information on the smoking status of people who had acute MI and analyzed the effects on nonsmokers. Seo and Torabi (2007) limited their study to acute MI patients who were nonsmokers, so observed decreases in acute MI are due to decreases in secondhand-smoke exposure. Pell et al. (2008) measured serum cotinine in nonsmokers, so they could draw conclusions about changes in secondhand-smoke exposure at the time of implementation of the ban rather than having to study the effect of the implementation of a smoking ban itself.

The relationship between smoking bans and decreases in air concentrations of secondhand smoke depends on the concentration of secondhand smoke in the air before the ban, the extent of the ban, and how well the ban is enforced and complied with. None of the key publications, however, contains information on the duration or pattern of exposure of individuals to secondhand smoke. That is, there is no information on how long or how often individuals were exposed before or after implementation of the smoking bans. For example, it is not known whether individuals were exposed to high concentrations sporadically for short periods or to low concentrations more consistently or both. Without that information, the committee could not determine whether acute exposures were triggering acute coronary events, chronic exposures were causing continuing damage that eventually resulted in acute coronary events, or a combination of chronic damage and acute exposure led to acute coronary events.

Although many of the key publications do not contain air-monitoring or biomarker data to assess the changes in secondhand smoke after ban implementation, other publications on the implementation of smoking bans, either in the regions examined in the key studies or in other regions, show that secondhand smoke decreases after implementation of a ban (see Chapter 2), and the committee concluded that generally the implementation of a smoking ban is associated with decreased air concentrations of secondhand smoke. Secondhand smoke reductions in the venues covered by the bans typically ranged from 50 to 90%. In addition, Pell et al. (2008) did measure serum cotinine in all acute MI cases reported and found that exposures decreased after implementation of a smoking ban.

There is information on compliance and enforcement of the eight smoking bans examined in the 11 key studies. Available data indicate compliance or a decrease in markers of secondhand smoke after the implementation of smoking bans in general but not for the specific study populations in the key publications in Italy (Gallus et al., 2006; Gorini et al., 2005; Valente et al., 2007), New York state (CDC, 2004, 2007; RTI International, 2004), and Scotland (Haw and Gruer, 2007; Menzies et al., 2006; Pell et al., 2008; Semple et al., 2007a, 2007b). Although no data on air sampling could be found for Helena, Montana; Pueblo, Colorado; and Saskatoon, Canada, data indicated a high degree of compliance with the smoking bans in those locations (Bartecchi et al., 2006; Lemstra et al., 2008; Sargent et al., 2004). There is no information on compliance, enforcement, or air monitoring for secondhand-smoke markers in Monroe County, Indiana. In contrast, air monitoring in Bowling Green, Ohio (Akbar-Khanzadeh et al., 2004) indicated that the magnitude of the decrease in secondhand-smoke markers in air was related to characteristics of the smoking restrictions. The concentration of secondhand-smoke–related compounds was lower in nonsmoking restaurants than in restaurants that permitted smoking in separate rooms.

On the basis of those data, the committee concludes that, with the exception of some establishments in Bowling Green, Ohio, the smoking bans evaluated in the key studies appear to have resulted in a large decrease in potential exposure to secondhand smoke. Decreases in acute MIs were seen in the two studies that evaluated effects only in nonsmokers (Pell et al., 2008; Seo and Torabi, 2007). Given those two facts, decreases in secondhand-smoke exposure likely contribute to the decreases in acute MIs after implementation of smoking bans seen in the studies that looked at the overall population (smokers and nonsmokers). The portion of the decrease in acute MIs that can be attributed specifically to changes in secondhand-smoke concentration, however, cannot be determined on the basis of the available data.

Outcomes

The key studies varied on the outcomes they examined. Some assessed changes in morbidity, others mortality, and others both. Morbidity and mortality from acute coronary events should be used as outcomes in considering the effect of a smoking ban. For mortality, ideally there would be autopsy confirmation of all deaths that might be due to acute coronary events; however, the larger the study, the less feasible that is. Short of that, medical records and other information could be reviewed independently to confirm the cause of death (not only for those coded as acute coronary events but for those not so coded but possibly acute coronary events nonetheless). For morbidity, there should be independent clinical confirmation, through review of medical charts and perhaps other information, that cases meet standardized criteria, such as those recommended by the World Health Organization (WHO) or others that take into consideration electrocardiography, biomarkers of cardiac damage, and pain. It is necessary, in the case of both mortality and morbidity, that *International Classification of Diseases (ICD)* guidelines be followed rigorously in identifying underlying causes of death and morbidity as opposed to merely abstracting the bottom line on the hospital discharge or the death certificate.

Surveillance studies rely heavily on the use of a standardized system for classification of diseases, *ICD*, issued by WHO. Most countries use that system in connection with hospitalizations as well as deaths. The United States, uniquely, uses a modification of the system, the *ICD-Clinical Modification (ICD-CM)*, to classify diagnostic information from medical records and for medical reimbursement. *ICD-CM* is more detailed, using an additional (fifth) coding digit. The *ICD* system is revised about every 10 years, and both *ICD-9* and *ICD-10* were in use in some countries in the key studies under review.[1]

Regardless of whether *ICD-9* or *ICD-10* is used, physicians and others typically list all causes of death and list the underlying cause of death last on the death certificate.[2] Regardless of the *ICD* code, that is often done incorrectly; coders using death certificates for gathering statistics are directed in the *ICD* rules to select the listed underlying cause of death only if it could have given rise to all the other conditions listed as among the causes of death. Otherwise, they are to determine a logical sequence of events that could have led to death and select the underlying cause of the sequence, disregarding "ill-defined conditions." In that respect, a change between *ICD-9* and *ICD-10* is of potential relevance to this review: in *ICD-10*, for the first time, the diagnosis "cardiac arrest, unspecified," I46.9, is regarded as ill-defined. In addition, what was a single code for acute MI in *ICD-9* (410) is expanded in *ICD-10* to six codes (I21.0–I21.4 and I21.9) that specify the site of MI. According to an analysis by the National Center for Health Statistics, the switch from *ICD-9* to *ICD-10* resulted in small but significant decreases in coding of cause of death as heart diseases in

---

[1] *ICD-10* endorsement by WHO in 1990 was followed by implementation at different times by different countries (WHO, 2009). According to the National Center for Health Statistics (National Center for Health Statistics, 2009), in the United States as of January 1, 1999, *ICD-10* has been used to code and classify mortality data from death certificates, and the U.S. Department of Health and Human Services has proposed regulations to replace *ICD-9-CM* codes with *ICD-10-CM* codes sets for health-care diagnoses and procedures as of October 1, 2011 (HHS, 2008). *ICD-10* codes were in use in the study in Saskatoon (Lemstra et al., 2008).

[2] WHO defines the underlying cause of death as the disease or injury that initiated the train of events that led directly to death or the circumstances of the accident or violence that produced the fatal injury.

general and acute MI in particular in the United States (Anderson et al., 2001); reporting of deaths as due to acute MI decreased by 10% in England and Wales (Griffiths et al., 2004) and decreased by 0.6% in Spain (Cirera Suarez et al., 2006).

Classification of deaths as acute coronary events on death certificates, regardless of whether *ICD-9* or *ICD-10* is used, poses general methodologic issues. On the one hand, a number of investigators have found that the numbers of such diagnoses are quite consistent over time (Goldacre et al., 2003; Mahonen et al., 1997; Pajunen et al., 2005). On the other hand, it was found in Finland that there was considerable variation among geographic areas and levels of care (for example, in local versus central hospitals) (Mahonen et al., 1997). Of more concern is the overall accuracy of physician-based determinations of cause of death in the absence of autopsies and the very low rate of autopsies performed, particularly in the United States (Kircher et al., 1985). Specifically, for deaths from acute MI, a hospital-based autopsy case series identified substantial discrepancies (48% were missed) between autopsy-proven diagnoses and death certificates (Ravakhah, 2006). A study in Australia also identified high rates of missed cases of acute coronary events in the absence of autopsy (Nashelsky and Lawrence, 2003). In considering the effect of such misdiagnoses in the 11 key studies, however, differences in accuracy over time or between locations (for example, between the study county and a comparison county) would be of most concern.

The diagnosis of acute coronary events at hospital discharge can also be problematic. The switch from *ICD-9* to *ICD-10* changed how repeated hospitalizations are coded, that is, whether a person who was admitted to the hospital with a diagnosis of an acute coronary event multiple times during the course of a study would be counted multiple times in the study. Counting multiple admissions for the same person's acute coronary events as though the admissions were of different persons might bias findings. *ICD-9* classifies the diagnosis according to the first or later visit for treatment of a particular MI on the basis of the site of the MI (for example, *ICD-9* 410.12 is the code for acute MI; other anterior wall; subsequent episode of care). *ICD-10* uses the term subsequent to refer to an MI within 4 weeks of a previous one regardless of the site.

In general, multiple studies have demonstrated that there are inaccuracies in the diagnosis of acute coronary events in medical records. A recent ecologic study in Texas found that only 401 of 496 cases of "definite myocardial infarction" met diagnostic criteria[3] for acute MI developed by the

---

[3] The criteria are based on electrocardiograms, cardiac enzymes, and cardiac pain as recorded in medical records.

Cardiovascular Community Surveillance Program (CCSP) (Pladevall et al., 1996).

To complicate the issue, there have been other changes in diagnostic criteria for acute coronary events over the past decade. Serial measures of biomarkers of cardiac damage have been incorporated into the revised 2003 case definition from the American Heart Association (AHA) and a number of international associations (Luepker et al., 2003). Assays that measure serum concentrations of two isoforms of cardiac troponin, cardiac troponin I (cTnI) and cardiac troponin T (cTnT), are now used in the case definition of acute coronary events.[4] Those assays are the most specific clinically available markers of acute coronary events. In relation to the key studies reviewed by the committee that only changes in diagnostic criteria that occurred during the timeframe of the study would affect the results of the study, and would only be relevant to studies that compared the same region before and after a smoking ban. All the key studies compare acute MIs before and after the ban, and the timeframes of all but two of the key studies (Barone-Adesi et al., 2006; Pell et al., 2008) include 2003, the time at which the case definition changed. Three of the studies include comparison populations (Lemstra et al., 2008; Pell et al., 2008; Sargent et al., 2004), and analyses with the comparison population would not be affected by the change in diagnostic criteria. It should be noted that a recent study showed that, compared with the earlier 1994 WHO MONICA (Multinational Monitoring of Trends and Determinants in Cardiovascular Disease) definition, the 2003 AHA case definition would increase the diagnosis of acute coronary events substantially (by 62–84%) if serum troponin were measured with sensitive assays (Kavsak et al., 2006). The changes in the criteria for an acute MI would be expected to increase reporting of acute MIs in later years, making a decrease in events after the smoking ban more difficult to detect. Despite that potential difficulty in detecting the decrease, the studies that looked at acute MI over time observed significant decreases (Bartecchi et al., 2006; CDC, 2009; Cesaroni et al., 2008; Juster et al., 2007; Khuder et al., 2007; Vasselli et al., 2008).

Time to Effect

The issue of the interval between an intervention (implementation of a smoking ban) and a change in the rate of acute coronary events is one of the questions included in the charge to the committee (Question 5) and is

---

[4] Assays have been developed for both cTnI and cTnT. Both are used to indicate myocardial damage. In this report, the committee uses the term *serum troponin* when discussing the assays in general but the term used by the authors of a publication when discussing the results of a specific study.

relevant to the committee's judgment as to the plausibility of a relationship between exposure to secondhand smoke and acute coronary events. The 11 publications differ in the followup time for acute MI. The shortest followup period is 2 months, in one of the Italian reports that demonstrated risk reductions after implementation of a ban (Vasselli et al., 2008). Other studies have looked at up to 6 months after a ban (Barone-Adesi et al., 2006; Sargent et al., 2004), between 6 months and 1 year (Cesaroni et al., 2008; Lemstra et al., 2008; Pell et al., 2008), and from more than 1 to 3 years (Bartecchi et al., 2006; CDC, 2009; Juster et al., 2007; Khuder et al., 2007; Seo and Torabi, 2007). Table 7-2 presents the periods examined in the publications and the risk reductions associated with them. As can be seen from that table, a small decrease in acute MIs—6.4% from the previous year and an estimated 13.1% from what was expected on the basis of linear regression (relative risk, 0.87; 95% confidence interval [CI], 0.84–0.93)—occurred as early as 2 months after implementation in Italy (Vasselli et al., 2008). According to Table 7-2, although there are many

TABLE 7-2 Followup Periods of Studies (listed from shortest to longest followup)

Publication (Region)	Followup Period[a]	Decrease in Admission Rates
Vasselli et al., 2008 (Four regions in Italy)[b]	0–2 months	6.4% decrease from 2004 to 2005 13.1% decrease (estimated) from expected based on linear regression (RR, 0.87; 95% CI, 0.84–0.93)
Sargent et al., 2004 (Helena, Montana)	0–6 months	40% decrease in average monthly admissions (from 40 to 24; 95% CI, decrease of 0.3–31.7%)
Barone-Adesi, 2006 (Piedmont region, Italy)[b]	0–5 months	11% decrease in those under 60 years old (RR, 0.89; 95% CI, 0.81–0.98) in February–June 2004
Pell et al., 2008 (Scotland)	0–10 months	17% decrease (95% CI, 16–18%) after implementation of smoking ban
Cesaroni et al., 2008 (Rome, Italy)[b]	0–12 months[c]	11% decrease in 35- to 64-year-olds (RR, 0.89; 95% CI, 0.85–0.93); 8% decrease in 65- to 74-year-olds (RR, 0.92; 95% CI, 0.88–0.97)

TABLE 7-2 Continued

Publication (Region)	Followup Period[a]	Decrease in Admission Rates
Lemstra et al., 2008 (Saskatoon, Canada)	0–12 months	13% decrease (rate ratio, 0.87; 95% CI, 0.84–0.90)
Khuder et al., 2007 (Bowling Green, Ohio)[d]	9–21 months	39% decrease in annual admission rates (95% CI, 33–45%) in 2002 (includes 2 months without ordinance)[e]
Bartecchi et al., 2006 (Pueblo, Colorado)	0–18 months	27% decrease in hospitalizations (acute MIs/100,000 person-years) (RR, 0.73; 95% CI, 0.63–0.85)
Seo and Torabi, 2007 (Monroe County, Indiana)	0–22 months	70% decrease in 2-year admissions (from 17 to 5 cases; decrease of 12 cases, 95% CI, 2.81–21.19)
Juster et al., 2007 (New York state)	5–17 months[f]	8% (estimated) fewer admissions in 2004 than expected with just local smoking bans implemented; 19% (estimated) fewer admissions in 2004 than expected if prior smoking bans had not been in effect
CDC, 2009 (Pueblo, Colorado)[g]	18–36 months	41% decrease (RR, 0.59; 95% CI, 0.49–0.70)
Khuder et al., 2007 (Bowling Green, Ohio)[d]	34–39 months	47% decrease in admission rates (95% CI, 41–55%)

Abbreviations: CI, confidence interval; MI, myocardial infarction; RR, relative risk.

[a] Period for which data were analyzed. Implementation of ban is at month zero. All periods are expressed in months. For some regions the ban was implemented for a part of a month. In those cases the exact dates of the study are footnoted.

[b] The four regions analyzed by Vasselli et al. (2008)—Piedmont, Friuli–Venezia–Giulia, Latium, Campania—contain areas analyzed by Barone-Adesi et al. (2006) and Cesaroni et al. (2008).

[c] Smoking ban was not implemented until January 10, 2005, so followup period is actually 10 days less than 1 year.

[d] Khuder et al. (2007) reported results at two times. Data were not analyzed for first 6 months after ban was implemented, to allow time for enforcement and compliance.

[e] Significant decrease in trend (parameter representing change in series level, $\omega = -1.69$; $p = 0.04$) in monthly series rate starting 7 months after full implementation and enforcement (November 2002).

[f] Smoking ban was implemented July 24, 2003, so the followup period is actually from 5 months and 7 days to 17 months and 6 days.

[g] Same study population as Bartecchi et al. (2006).

uncertainties in and variability among the different studies, the decreases in general appear to be larger with longer followup periods. The committee did not conduct any analyses to assess whether there are differences with different periods. However, data presented to the committee by Dr. Stanton Glantz demonstrated a relationship between study length and magnitude of risk reduction (personal communication, Stanton Glantz, University of California, San Francisco School of Medicine, January 30, 2009).[5]

The time between an intervention and its effect is difficult to determine when there is no precise date of the intervention. As discussed previously for smoking bans, many activities occur before and around the time of implementation of legislation. Those activities could result in changes in smoking behaviors before the ban was implemented, blurring the timing of the intervention (for example, whether the intervention occurs when the legislation is implemented or whether the intervention occurs when a public discussion about a ban begins). Improved compliance with the ban over time or use of a phase-in period could also delay the effective date of the full intervention, further blurring its timing.

Some of the studies indicate that an effect was seen as early as within 2 months of the implementation of a smoking ban (Vasselli et al., 2008). The majority of the studies show effects within months of implementation. However, given the blurred timing of the interventions and the numerous differences among the studies—such as in the characteristics of the smoking bans, in the implementation of smoking restrictions or bans before implementation of the bans under study, and in background rates of smoking and acute MIs—the key intervention studies do not provide strong evidence on which to establish a more precise time between an intervention and a decrease in risk of acute MI.

Plausibility

As the key studies showing reductions in acute MIs after implementation of smoking bans were published, some skepticism was expressed as to the believability or likelihood of the effects, whether a detectable change in heart attacks could possibly be associated with banning smoking in public places and offices, and whether the magnitude of the effect could be as high as seen in some of the studies. The committee considered two aspects of plausibility: the biologic plausibility of the effect and the plausibility of the magnitude of the effect.

---

[5] The analysis presented to the committee was published after the committee's report entered review (Lightwood and Glantz, 2009).

Biologic Plausibility of an Effect

The committee reviewed the pathophysiologic data on secondhand smoke and its components to evaluate whether there are biologic modes of action by which secondhand smoke could have cardiovascular events and, in particular, whether the absence of exposure to secondhand smoke could be associated with a decrease in acute MIs. Chapter 3 reviews the effects of secondhand smoke and its components on the cardiovascular system. Experimental studies have been conducted in humans, in animals, and in cell preparations to look at end points that are related to cardiovascular disease. Experimental studies of secondhand smoke and some of its components, including particulate matter (PM), demonstrate that they exert substantial cardiovascular toxicity. The toxicologic effects include endothelial dysfunction, increased thrombosis, inflammation, and adversely affected plaque stability; all these phenomena are on the pathway to acute MI. The pathophysiologic results are consistent with the results of the key ecologic studies, especially the two studies that looked at effects in nonsmokers, which show the rate of acute MI decreasing with a decrease in secondhand-smoke exposure; however, the ecologic studies do not (and cannot) address timeframes of less than 1 month. The data support a role of secondhand smoke as a potential causative agent in acute coronary events, that is, they constitute evidence that it is biologically plausible for secondhand smoke to be a causative agent in cardiovascular disease and acute coronary events.

Plausibility of Magnitude of an Effect

When considering the plausibility of the magnitude of the effect, the committee looked at the effects seen in the studies that examined the effects of secondhand smoke and the implementation of smoking bans compared with studies that examined the effects of smoking, and with studies that examined the effects of PM in air pollution.

Comparison with Data on Smokers. One aspect of the plausibility of an effect of secondhand smoke that is often questioned is the size of the effect relative to the size of the effect of smoking, especially in light of the fact that smokers also inhale secondhand smoke. The epidemiologic studies reviewed in this report show a decrease of about 6–47% in the risk of acute MI after implementation of a smoking ban (Barone-Adesi et al., 2006; Bartecchi et al., 2006; CDC, 2009; Cesaroni et al., 2008; Juster et al., 2007; Khuder et al., 2007; Lemstra et al., 2008; Pell et al., 2008; Sargent et al., 2004; Seo and Torabi, 2007; Vasselli et al., 2008); an increase in the odds ratio (OR) of 1.24 (95% CI, 1.17–1.32) to 1.62 (95% CI, 1.45–1.81) for secondhand-smoke exposure for 1–7 hours/week and at least 22 hours/week, respectively, in the INTERHEART case–control study (Teo et al., 2006); and a nonsignificant OR of 1.19 (95% CI, 0.78–1.82) for the highest tertile of lifetime cumulative exposure compared with the lowest tertile of lifetime cumulative exposure (Stranges et al., 2006). It should be noted, however, that cumulative lifetime exposure may not be the appropriate exposure metric for the relationship between secondhand-smoke exposure and acute MI. In fact, the observed reduction in acute MI within a year of smoking bans indicates that recent exposure is more relevant. Such an interpretation is supported by the pathophysiologic responses to a 30-minute exposure to secondhand smoke (see Chapter 3). In the INTERHEART study (Teo et al., 2006), the OR for secondhand-smoke exposure (1.24–1.62, depending on the magnitude of exposure) can be compared to an overall OR for smoking of 2.95 (95% CI, 2.77–3.14). In that study, the OR for smoking ranged from 1.63 (95% CI, 1.45–1.82) for smoking one to nine cigarettes per day to 4.59 (95% CI, 4.21–5.00) for smoking 20 or more cigarettes per day. Regression analysis indicates that the risk of developing acute MI increases by 1.056 (95% CI, 1.05–1.06) for every additional cigarette smoked per day (Teo et al., 2006). Therefore, the increase in risk of acute MI associated with secondhand-smoke exposure in the case–control studies and the decrease in risk of acute MI seen after implementation of smoking bans are about the same or smaller than those seen with a low level of current smoking and substantially smaller than those seen with current heavy smoking. In looking at smoking cessation and the decrease in risks, the INTERHEART study showed that the risk of acute MI in those who quit smoking 1–3 years earlier decreased to 1.87 (95% CI, 1.55–2.24) and continued to decrease with time; some risk remained, however, even years after cessation smoking (Teo et al., 2006).

Comparison with Data on Particulate Matter in Air Pollution. PM is a major component of secondhand smoke (see Chapter 2). The composition of PM, including particle size, can affect its toxicity and is different between secondhand smoke and air pollution and between air pollution from different sources (Dockery, 2009). Both secondhand smoke and air pollution contain fine and ultrafine PM, so the committee conducted some analyses to compare the effects seen in the key studies with those seen in response to the PM in air pollution. Although the two types of PM differ in some characteristics, the committee concluded that there were enough similarities between the $PM_{2.5}$ (PM with an aerodynamic diameter of less than 2.5 μm) in secondhand smoke and that in ambient air pollution to warrant comparison of the magnitudes of the effects of the two. This is not done to estimate the number of people who would have cardiovascular effects because of the PM in secondhand smoke but rather serves as a "reality check" on the numbers that were seen in the key epidemiologic studies related to smoking bans.

The committee developed several scenarios of exposure to $PM_{2.5}$ concentrations that represent lower or higher exposures to secondhand smoke and estimated the increased risk of and attributable number of hospital admissions for heart failure and cardiovascular disease in a portion of the U.S. population on the basis of the scenarios (see Tables 7-3, 7-4, and 7-5). The estimates used data from Medicare, and so reflect effects only on those ages 65 years or older, are only for a subset of counties in the United States, and are based solely on the cardiovascular effects of PM. Therefore, the estimates do not represent the potential public-health impact of secondhand smoke but are provided to put the decreases in hospital admissions seen in the key studies that evaluated the effect of smoking bans in the context of the health effects of one of the constituents of secondhand smoke.

For each scenario, the committee calculated, on the basis of published data, the daily average concentration of ambient $PM_{2.5}$. One main source of the exposure data was the 16 Cities Study, in which about 100 people in each of 16 U.S. metropolitan areas wore two personal samplers (one at work for about 8 hours and one when "away from work," typically at home) that measured several components of secondhand smoke, including respirable particles (measured in that study as $PM_{3.5}$).[6] From the home samples in that study, there were 935 personal samples from people who reported that no one smoked in their homes and the measured nicotine concentrations were under 0.1 $\mu g/m^3$; they were exposed to respirable particles at an average of 18 $\mu g/m^3$. There were 372 samples from people who reported that they lived with smokers; they were exposed to an average of $PM_{3.5}$ at 44 $\mu g /m^3$. Those values agree well with PM measurements made in randomly selected homes in New York state, where average "respirable suspended particle" concentrations were 15 $\mu g/m^3$ and 44 $\mu g/m^3$ in non-smoking and smoking homes, respectively (Leaderer and Hammond, 1991). There were 768 samples from workers who reported that smoking was not allowed in their workplaces and the measured nicotine concentrations were under 0.1 $\mu g/m^3$. They were exposed to $PM_{3.5}$ at an average of 16 $\mu g/m^3$. The 355 workers who reported that smoking was allowed in their workplaces and who had observed someone smoking on the day of the sampling were exposed to $PM_{3.5}$ at an average of 50 $\mu g/m^3$.

The PM concentrations used for the various venues were as follows:

---

[6] Concentrations were compiled from the data used in Doses and Lung Burdens of Environmental Tobacco Smoke Constituents in Nonsmoking Workplaces (Gevecker Graves et al., 2000).

TABLE 7-3 Estimates of Increased Risk of Cardiovascular Disease and Annual Reduction in Hospital Admissions for Cardiovascular Disease with Changes in Particulate-Matter Exposures[a]

Exposure Scenario	Additional Exposure (Total Exposure), $\mu g/m^{3b}$	Increased Risk of Cardiovascular Disease[c] (Lower Estimate, Upper Estimate)	Annual Reduction in Hospital Admissions[d] (Lower Estimate, Upper Estimate)
Nonsmoking workplace, nonsmoking home (reference concentration, assuming 16 h at home, 17 $\mu g/m^3$)			
8 h at work; 15 h at home; 1 h at pub or bar	16.3 (33)	1.15 (0.73, 1.56)	10,470 (6,622, 14,185)
8 h at work; 12 h at home; 4 h at pub or bar	64.0 (81)	4.54 (2.88, 6.14)	41,942 (26,362, 57,170)
8 h at work; 14.5 h at home; 1.5 h at bowling alley	3.0 (20)	0.21 (0.13, 0.28)	1,897 (1,202, 2,566)
8 h at work; 6 h at home; 2 h at pub or bar	76.0 (93)	5.40 (3.42, 7.30)	50,021 (31,389, 68,286)
Smoking workplace, nonsmoking home (reference concentration, assuming 16 h at home, 17 $\mu g/m^3$)			
8 h at work; 15 h at home; 1 h at pub or bar	27.6 (45)	1.96 (1.24, 2.65)	17,843 (11,269, 24,210)
8 h at work; 12 h at home; 4 h at pub or bar	75.3 (92)	5.35 (3.39, 7.23)	49,570 (31,109, 67,665)
8 h at work; 14.5 h at home; 1.5 h at bowling alley	14.3 (31)	1.01 (0.64, 1.37)	9,201 (5,821, 12,464)
8 h at work; 6 h at home; 2 h at pub or bar	87.5 (105)	6.21 (3.94, 8.40)	57,828 (36,233, 79,060)
Nonsmoking workplace, smoking home (reference concentration, assuming 16 h at home, 35 $\mu g/m^3$)			
8 h at work; 15 h at home; 1 h at pub or bar	14.5 (50)	1.03 (0.65, 1.39)	9,336 (5,906, 12,647)
8 h at work; 12 h at home; 4 h at pub or bar	59.0 (94)	4.19 (2.66, 5.66)	38,596 (24,275, 52,576)
8 h at work; 14.5 h at home; 1.5 h at bowling alley	0.7 (36)	0.05 (0.03, 0.06)	427 (271, 578)
8 h at work; 6 h at home; 2 h at pub or bar	64.7 (100)	4.59 (2.91, 6.21)	42,389 (26,640, 57,784)

TABLE 7-3 Continued

Exposure Scenario	Additional Exposure (Total Exposure), $\mu g/m^{3b}$	Increased Risk of Cardiovascular Disease[c] (Lower Estimate, Upper Estimate)	Annual Reduction in Hospital Admissions[d] (Lower Estimate, Upper Estimate)
Smoking workplace, smoking home (reference concentration, assuming 16 h at home, 35 $\mu g/m^3$)			
8 h at work; 15 h at home; 1 h at pub or bar	25.8 (61)	1.83 (1.16, 2.48)	16,701 (10,549, 22,655)
8 h at work; 12 h at home; 4 h at pub or bar	70.3 (105)	4.99 (3.17, 6.75)	46,197 (29,012, 63,021)
8 h at work; 14.5 h at home; 1.5 h at bowling alley	12.0 (47)	0.85 (0.54, 1.15)	7,720 (4,885, 10,454)
8 h at work; 6 h at home; 2 h at pub or bar	76.0 (111)	5.40 (3.42, 7.30)	50,021 (31,389, 68,286)

[a] Committee calculated changes in particulate-matter exposures for different exposure scenarios and estimated corresponding changes in risk of cardiovascular-disease admissions due to those changes and corresponding reductions in annual hospital admissions in 204 largest urban counties on basis of hospital admissions data from U.S. Medicare database.

[b] Daily exposure to particulate matter in addition to the reference concentration.

[c] Increased risk calculated by using relative-risk estimate of 0.71 (95% CI, 0.45–0.96; Lag = 0) per 10-$\mu g/m^3$ increase in $PM_{2.5}$. Increased risk estimate is based on data from Peng et al. (2008).

[d] Changes in number of hospital admissions is based on Medicare data from 204 largest urban counties, which has a total of 11.5 million Medicare enrollees.

pubs and bars,[7] 400 $\mu g/m^3$ (Akbar-Khanzadeh et al., 2004; CDC, 2004; Ellingsen et al., 2006; Lofroth and Lazaridis, 1986; Semple et al., 2007b; Valente et al., 2007); restaurants,[8] 200 $\mu g/m^3$ (Alpert et al., 2007; Ellingsen et al., 2006; Valente et al., 2007); bowling alleys, 60 $\mu g/m^3$ (CDC, 2004); pool halls and video-game arcades, 150 $\mu g/m^3$ (CDC, 2004); bingo parlors, 400 $\mu g/m^3$ (CDC, 2004; Kado et al., 1991); casinos, 200 $\mu g/m^3$ (Kado et al., 1991); and nonsmoking establishments or venues, 20 $\mu g/m^3$.

Total average 24-hour $PM_{2.5}$ exposure was estimated by assuming

---

[7] Pubs in Europe were deemed most like bars in the United States, so data from those venues were combined in a single category named "pubs and bars."

[8] In Europe, "bars" typically serve food, so the committee assumed that European bars are like restaurants in the United States (which might or might not have bar sections) and combined them in a single "restaurants" category.

TABLE 7-4 Estimates of Increased Risk of Ischemic Heart Disease and Annual Reduction in Hospital Admissions for Ischemic Heart Disease with Changes in Particulate-Matter Exposures[a]

Exposure Scenario	Additional Exposure (Total Exposure), $\mu g/m^{3b}$	Increased Risk of Heart Failure[c] (Lower Estimate, Upper Estimate)	Annual Reduction in Hospital Admissions[d] (Lower Estimate, Upper Estimate)
Nonsmoking workplace, nonsmoking home (reference concentration, assuming 16 h at home, 17 $\mu g/m^3$)			
8 h at work; 15 h at home; 1 h at pub or bar	16.3 (33)	2.19 (1.23, 2.94)	5,498 (3,570, 7,399)
8 h at work; 12 h at home; 4 h at pub or bar	64.0 (81)	8.64 (5.63, 11.58)	22,368 (14,360, 30,442)
8 h at work; 14.5 h at home; 1.5 h at bowling alley	3.0 (20)	0.40 (0.26, 0.54)	992 (646, 1,331)
8 h at work; 6 h at home; 2 h at pub or bar	76.0 (93)	10.26 (6.69, 13.76)	26,781 (17,144, 36,553)
Smoking workplace, nonsmoking home (reference concentration, assuming 16 h at home, 17 $\mu g/m^3$)			
8 h at work; 15 h at home; 1 h at pub or bar	27.6 (45)	3.72 (2.43, 4.99)	9,404 (6,090, 12,689)
8 h at work; 12 h at home; 4 h at pub or bar	75.3 (92)	10.17 (6.63, 13.64)	26,534 (16,989, 36,210)
8 h at work; 14.5 h at home; 1.5 h at bowling alley	14.3 (31)	1.93 (1.26, 2.59)	4,829 (3,137, 6,495)
8 h at work; 6 h at home; 2 h at pub or bar	87.5 (105)	11.81 (7.70, 15.84)	31,078 (19,840, 42,535)
Nonsmoking workplace, smoking home (reference concentration, assuming 16 h at home, 35 $\mu g/m^3$)			
8 h at work; 15 h at home; 1 h at pub or bar	14.5 (50)	1.96 (1.28, 2.62)	4,900 (3,183, 6,591)
8 h at work; 12 h at home; 4 h at pub or bar	59.0 (94)	7.97 (5.19, 10.68)	20,550 (13,209, 27,935)
8 h at work; 14.5 h at home; 1.5 h at bowling alley	0.7 (36)	0.09 (0.06, 0.12)	223 (145, 299)
8 h at work; 6 h at home; 2 h at pub or bar	64.7 (100)	8.73 (5.69, 11.70)	22,611 (14,514, 30,778)
Smoking workplace, smoking home (reference concentration, assuming 16 h at home, 35 $\mu g/m^3$)			
8 h at work; 15 h at home; 1 h at pub or bar	25.8 (61)	3.49 (2.27, 4.68)	8,797 (5,699, 11,865)
8 h at work; 12 h at home; 4 h at pub or bar	70.3 (105)	9.50 (6.19, 12.73)	24,688 (15,826, 33,651)

TABLE 7-4 Continued

Exposure Scenario	Additional Exposure (Total Exposure), $\mu g/m^{3b}$	Increased Risk of Heart Failure[c] (Lower Estimate, Upper Estimate)	Annual Reduction in Hospital Admissions[d] (Lower Estimate, Upper Estimate)
8 h at work; 14.5 h at home; 1.5 h at bowling alley	12.0 (47)	1.62 (1.06, 2.17)	4,048 (2,631, 5,443)
8 h at work; 6 h at home; 2 h at pub or bar	76.0 (111)	10.26 (6.69, 13.76)	26,781 (17,144, 36,553)

[a] Committee calculated changes in particulate-matter exposures for different exposure scenarios and estimated corresponding changes in risk of ischemic heart disease due to those changes and corresponding reductions in annual hospital admissions in 204 largest urban counties on basis of hospital admissions data from U.S. Medicare database.

[b] Daily exposure to particulate matter in addition to the reference concentration.

[c] Increased risk calculated by using a relative-risk estimate of 0.25 (95% CI, –0.12 to 0.62; Lag = 0) per 10-$\mu g/m^3$ increase in $PM_{2.5}$. That increased risk estimate is based on data from Peng et al. (2008).

[d] Changes in number of hospital admissions is based on Medicare data from 204 largest urban counties, which has a total of 11.5 million Medicare enrollees.

that people spent 8 hours at work, a varied number of hours in the different public venues, and the remaining 9–16 hours at home or, if they were retired, a varied number of hours in the different public venues and the remaining hours at home. In its calculations, the committee also assumed that smoking bans did not affect home exposures. Reductions in 24-hour average $PM_{2.5}$ exposures (from pre–smoking ban concentrations in workplaces and public venues) were calculated separately for those living with smokers and those who lived in homes without any smoking (see Tables 7-3, 7-4, and 7-5).

The committee assumed that the $PM_{2.5}$ concentrations correlate with the concentrations of secondhand-smoke exposure in various venues. For each scenario, it calculated the difference in 24-hour average $PM_{2.5}$ exposure that would result from smoking bans for those who lived with smokers and for those who lived in smoke-free homes. The committee used data on changes in daily exposure to $PM_{2.5}$ and cardiovascular diseases from epidemiologic studies of the Medicare population (which includes only people at least 65 years old) and extracted the percentage increases in the risk of emergency hospital admissions for all cardiovascular diseases (Table 7-3), ischemic heart disease (Table 7-4), and heart failure (Table 7-5) associated with a 10-$\mu g/m^3$ reduction in $PM_{2.5}$ (Peng et al., 2008). For example, Peng et al. (2008) reported that, for the population over 65 years old living in

TABLE 7-5 Estimates of Increased Risk of Heart Failure and Annual Reduction in Hospital Admissions for Heart Failure with Changes in Particulate-Matter Exposures[a]

Exposure Scenario	Additional Exposure (Total Exposure), $\mu g/m^{3}$ [b]	Increased Risk of Heart Failure[c] (Lower Estimate, Upper Estimate)	Annual Reduction in Hospital Admissions[d] (Lower Estimate, Upper Estimate)
Nonsmoking workplace, nonsmoking home (reference concentration, assuming 16 h at home, 17 $\mu g/m^3$)			
8 h at work; 15 h at home; 1 h at pub or bar	16.3 (33)	2.19 (1.23, 2.94)	5,498 (3,570, 7,399)
8 h at work; 12 h at home; 4 h at pub or bar	64.0 (81)	8.64 (5.63, 11.58)	22,368 (14,360, 30,442)
8 h at work; 14.5 h at home; 1.5 h at bowling alley	3.0 (20)	0.40 (0.26, 0.54)	992 (646, 1,331)
8 h at work; 6 h at home; 2 h at pub or bar	76.0 (93)	10.26 (6.69, 13.76)	26,781 (17,144, 36,553)
Smoking workplace, nonsmoking home (reference concentration, assuming 16 h at home, 17 $\mu g/m^3$)			
8 h at work; 15 h at home; 1 h at pub or bar	27.6 (45)	3.72 (2.43, 4.99)	9,404 (6,090, 12,689)
8 h at work; 12 h at home; 4 h at pub or bar	75.3 (92)	10.17 (6.63, 13.64)	26,534 (16,989, 36,210)
8 h at work; 14.5 h at home; 1.5 h at bowling alley	14.3 (31)	1.93 (1.26, 2.59)	4,829 (3,137, 6,495)
8 h at work; 6 h at home; 2 h at pub or bar	87.5 (105)	11.81 (7.70, 15.84)	31,078 (19,840, 42,535)
Nonsmoking workplace, smoking home (reference concentration, assuming 16 h at home, 35 $\mu g/m^3$)			
8 h at work; 15 h at home; 1 h at pub or bar	14.5 (50)	1.96 (1.28, 2.62)	4,900 (3,183, 6,591)
8 h at work; 12 h at home; 4 h at pub or bar	59.0 (94)	7.97 (5.19, 10.68)	20,550 (13,209, 27,935)
8 h at work; 14.5 h at home; 1.5 h at bowling alley	0.7 (36)	0.09 (0.06, 0.12)	223 (145, 299)
8 h at work; 6 h at home; 2 h at pub or bar	64.7 (100)	8.73 (5.69, 11.70)	22,611 (14,514, 30,778)
Smoking workplace, smoking home (reference concentration, assuming 16 h at home, 35 $\mu g/m^3$)			
8 h at work; 15 h at home; 1 h at pub or bar	25.8 (61)	3.49 (2.27, 4.68)	8,797 (5,699, 11,865)
8 h at work; 12 h at home; 4 h at pub or bar	70.3 (105)	9.50 (6.19, 12.73)	24,688 (15,826, 33,651)

TABLE 7-5 Continued

Exposure Scenario	Additional Exposure (Total Exposure), $\mu g/m^{3b}$	Increased Risk of Heart Failure[c] (Lower Estimate, Upper Estimate)	Annual Reduction in Hospital Admissions[d] (Lower Estimate, Upper Estimate)
8 h at work; 14.5 h at home; 1.5 h at bowling alley	12.0 (47)	1.62 (1.06, 2.17)	4,048 (2,631, 5,443)
8 h at work; 6 h at home; 2 h at pub or bar	76.0 (111)	10.26 (6.69, 13.76)	26,781 (17,144, 36,553)

[a] Committee calculated changes in particulate-matter exposures for different exposure scenarios and estimated corresponding changes in risk of heart failure due to those changes and corresponding reductions in annual hospital admissions in 204 largest urban counties on basis of hospital admissions data from U.S. Medicare database.

[b] Daily exposure to particulate matter in addition to the reference concentration.

[c] Increased risk calculated by using relative-risk estimate of 1.35 (95% CI, 0.88–1.81; Lag = 0) per 10-$\mu g/m^3$ increase in $PM_{2.5}$. That increased risk estimate is based on data from Peng et al. (2008).

[d] Changes in number of hospital admissions is based on Medicare data from 204 largest urban counties, which has a total of 11.5 million Medicare enrollees.

the largest 204 urban counties in the United States (which contain about 12 million people, or one-fourth of the U.S. population), a daily increase in ambient $PM_{2.5}$ of 10 $\mu g/m^3$ is associated with an increase in the number of emergency hospital admissions for cardiovascular disease on a given day of 0.71% (95% CI, 0.45–0.96%). The corresponding increase in the number of admissions for ischemic heart disease is 0.25% (95% CI, –0.12 to 0.62%) and for heart failure 1.35% (95% CI, 0.88–1.81%).

The committee applied the calculated percentage increase in risk to the daily changes in $PM_{2.5}$ that occurred from secondhand-smoke exposures outside the home, that is, when a person worked where smoking occurred or spent time in a venue with smoking, such as a restaurant, bar, or casino. For each scenario, two comparison populations were evaluated: those who did not live with smokers and those who lived with smokers. The baseline for each was no other secondhand-smoke exposure, that is, the experience under a strong smoking ban. For example, the first comparison group is a population of nonsmokers who work and live in a nonsmoking environment. They are exposed to a 24-hour average $PM_{2.5}$ of 17 $\mu g/m^3$. Without a smoking ban, their daily average $PM_{2.5}$ exposure might increase to 33 $\mu g/m^3$ if they spent 1 hour in a pub. By comparing the two populations, the committee found a decrease in daily average $PM_{2.5}$ exposure of 16

$\mu g/m^3$ as a result of the smoking ban.[9] That decrease is associated with an annual reduction in hospital admissions for all cardiovascular diseases of 10,470 in about 11.5 million Medicare enrollees or, extrapolated to the entire U.S. population, about 40,000 (see Table 7-3). Those estimates indicate that changes in individual PM exposure that would be expected after implementation of smoking bans would be expected to result in substantial reductions in hospital admissions, and this implies that the results seen in the 11 key studies are plausible. Although there is uncertainty in the risk estimates associated with PM, especially for ischemic heart disease, much of the uncertainty is a result of the low numbers of hospital admission per day (and the committee would not necessarily recommend looking at the effects of smoking bans with that method); the analyses are clearly consistent with the magnitude of effects observed in the smoking-ban studies and strengthen confidence in the validity of the studies.

Analytic Issues

The studies used different analytic approaches; the most common was to estimate rate ratios, that is, to divide an admission rate after implementation of a ban by the admission rate before the ban. Some studies also used regression models to estimate age- and sex-adjusted rates of acute coronary events from monthly time-series data. Many of the analyses did not adjust for seasonality although some used data from the same months before and after implementation of a ban to control for seasonal differences.

Statistical analyses should be planned a priori. All planned analyses should be conducted and their results reported, and they should account for seasonality. Some of the epidemiologic studies of smoking bans and acute cardiovascular diseases used "interrupted time-series analysis methods" to estimate the effect of smoking bans on rates of hospital admissions for cardiovascular diseases. Those studies specify a regression model that includes several terms to account for different types of temporal confounding (such as seasonality and underlying trends). As is common in epidemiologic analysis of observational data, the results might be sensitive to the specification of the regression model and, more specifically, to the extent of control of unmeasured temporal confounding.

In this section, the committee examines the sensitivity of the results to the specification of the regression model in "interrupted time-series analysis methods" used in the studies of the public-health implications of smoking bans. The committee constructed a data set by using Medicare billing claims data for a population of elderly people. It constructed county-level age-adjusted monthly hospital admission rates for acute MI for the period

---

[9] Note that an even greater decrease in $PM_{2.5}$ would be experienced by those who had worked where smoking was allowed.

1999–2006 for the same 62 New York counties analyzed by Juster et al. (2007). This analysis does not replicate that of Juster et al. but illustrates the effect that model choice can have on results.

The committee used a Poisson regression model in which the outcome is the monthly number of hospital admissions for a given age group; the committee considered three age groups: 65–74 years, 75–84 years, and 85 years and over. The model included the following covariates:

- The natural logarithm of the number of the monthly Medicare enrollees in each age group (offset).
- A linear time-trend variable (month) to quantify changes in treatment, population risk factors, and other secular trends.
- A binary variable to capture the main effect of the instantaneous change in rates of hospital admission at the time of the smoking-ban implementation (July 24, 2003); equal to zero before implementation and equal to 1 after implementation.
- The interaction between the binary variable (representing the ban) and time; this analysis allows predicted hospital admission rates to continue to decline (or increase) linearly with time after implementation.
- A county indicator to account for differences among counties in average rates of hospital admissions.
- Interactions between county and time to control for county-specific secular changes; this analysis allows each county to have its own predicted linear trend.
- Indicator variables of month of year to control for seasonality.

The committee assessed the sensitivity of the results to the regression model by using the following four scenarios:

Scenario 1 assumed that the underlying trend, common to all the counties, is linear for the entire period 1999–2006.

Scenario 2 assumed that the underlying trend, common to all the counties, is a spline with 3 degrees of freedom for the entire period 1999–2006.

Scenario 3 assumed that the underlying trend, common to all the counties, is linear for the entire period 1999–2006 (as in Scenario 1) but fitted the regression model to the data from before implementation of a smoking ban and predicted the outcome after implementation.

Scenario 4 assumed that the underlying trend, common to all the counties, is a spline with 3 degrees of freedom for the entire period 1999–2006 (as in Scenario 2) but fitted the regression model to the data from before implementation of a smoking ban and predicted the outcome after implementation.

Figures 7-1–7-4 show the observed admissions for acute MI and those predicted without the statewide smoking ban under Scenarios 1–4, respectively. Figure 7-5 shows the estimated underlying trend for the whole period when a spline with 3 degrees of freedom was used (Scenarios 2 and 4). Table 7-6 summarizes the point estimates, the 95% CIs, and the p-values of the main effect of the smoking ban and the interaction term between the smoking ban and the linear function of time. The committee estimated these quantities under two regression models defined under Scenarios 1 and 2, which use linear and spline trends, respectively. As can be seen in Table 7-6, the resulting estimate changed from 0.0338 (95% CI, 0.0038–0.057; p = 0.0272) with a linear trend to 0.0503 (95% CI, 0.0110–0.089; p = 0.0122) with a spline trend.

The difference in results between Figure 7-1 and Figure 7-2 depends on the assumption of linearity in the trend in rates of acute MI during the entire study period (Scenario 1). If the assumption of linearity is relaxed, the results change substantially because the committee is estimating the trend for the entire study period, that is, using data from before and after

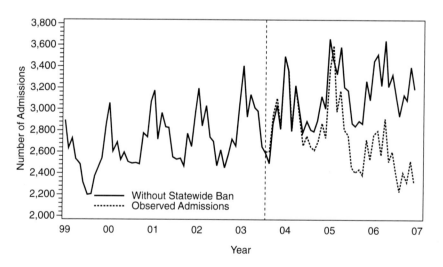

FIGURE 7-1 Observed admissions for acute MI and those predicted without statewide smoking ban on basis of Scenario 1. The dashed vertical line indicates when during 2003 the statewide ban was implemented.

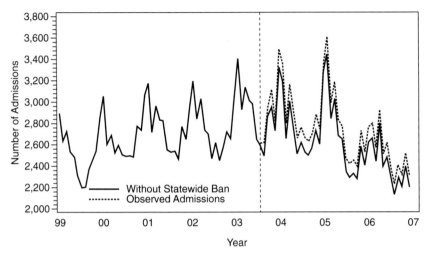

FIGURE 7-2 Observed admissions for acute MI and those predicted without state-wide smoking ban on basis of Scenario 2. The dashed vertical line indicates when during 2003 the statewide ban was implemented.

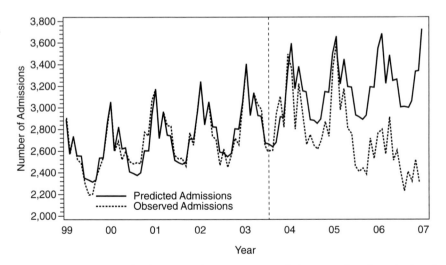

FIGURE 7-3 Observed admissions for acute MI and those predicted on basis of Scenario 3. The dashed vertical line indicates when during 2003 the statewide ban was implemented.

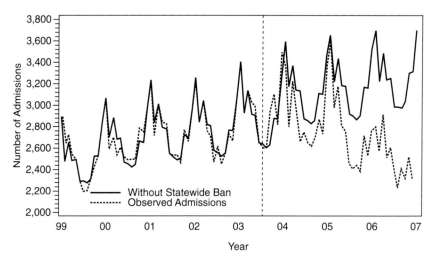

FIGURE 7-4 Observed admissions for acute MI and those predicted on basis of Scenario 4. The dashed vertical line indicates when during 2003 the statewide ban was implemented.

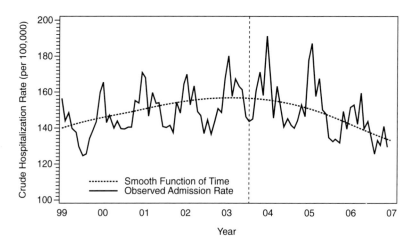

FIGURE 7-5 Crude acute MI hospitalization rate (per 100,000) with smooth function of time using 3 degrees of freedom. The dashed vertical line indicates when during 2003 the statewide ban was implemented.

TABLE 7-6 Summary of Point Estimates, 95% Confidence Intervals, and p-values of Main Effect of Smoking Ban and Interaction Term Between Smoking Ban and Linear Function of Time

	Estimate[a]	95% Confidence Interval		p-value
Acute MI scenario 1				
Statewide smoking ban	0.0338	0.0038	0.0537	0.0272
Statewide smoking ban by time interaction	–0.0077	–0.0094	–0.0059	<0.0001
Acute MI scenario 2				
Estimate of main effect of statewide smoking ban without statewide smoking ban by time interaction	0.0503	0.0110	0.0896	0.0122
Estimate of main effect of statewide smoking ban with statewide smoking ban by time interaction	0.0706	0.0288	0.1123	0.0009
Statewide smoking ban by time interaction	–0.0073	–0.0136	–0.009	0.0248

[a] Beta coefficient representing change in hospitalization rate over time after implementation of smoking ban.

implementation of a ban. Estimates of the trend (both linear and spline) based on only data from before the ban are less sensitive to the parametric specification of the trend. Another important assumption is in the interpretation of the results. In fitting a linear trend, the authors of all the studies assumed that any departure in the observed number of hospital admissions from the linear trend after implementation should be attributed entirely to the ban.

The committee did not explore which model and assumptions are most appropriate but presents this information to examine the effect of model choice. Given that model choice can affect the results substantially, it is important to discuss the rationale for and the sensitivity of the results to the choice of model in publications, especially for more statistically sophisticated analyses.

Publication Bias

The published studies all showed some statistically significant evidence that smoking bans reduced the risk of cardiovascular disease events. There is a possibility that if an investigation shows no reduction or a small reduction that is not statistically significant, the investigators will not be motivated to submit the results for publication or, if they do submit them, journal editors will consider such "negative studies" to be of low priority. Those considerations do not invalidate the published studies, but they suggest that a meta-analysis or quantitative estimate based on the published studies might overestimate the effects of smoking bans. The committee tried to identify and seek the results of all studies of the effects of smoking bans on the incidence of cardiovascular disease events. It searched CRISP and ClinicalTrials.gov to determine whether other studies of the effects of smoking bans on acute coronary events had been funded or approved and never published, and it found none. The National Association of City and County Health Officials Web site was also searched to determine whether other studies had been initiated, and the committee requested information from the Centers for Disease Control and Prevention and AHA on other studies that were under way or had been conducted and never published; no such studies were identified. There is still the possibility that studies showing no association were conducted but not published; this would bias the data toward there being an association between secondhand-smoke exposure or smoking bans and acute coronary events.

WEIGHT OF EVIDENCE FROM KEY STUDIES

The 11 studies reviewed in this chapter show remarkable consistency: all were observational studies that used different analyses and showed decreases in the rate of acute MI after implementation of eight smoking bans. Those decreases ranged from about 6 to 47%, depending on the study and the analysis. That consistency in the direction of change gave the committee confidence that smoking bans result in a real decrease in the rate of acute MIs.

Apart from their consistency, most studies drew conclusions that appear to be stronger than the data and analyses warranted. Some researchers have combined the results of the studies with meta-analytic methods to provide a point estimate of the decrease and an associated standard error (Glantz, 2008; Richiardi et al., 2009). The committee concluded that there are too many differences among the studies to have confidence in such a point estimate based on combining results of the different studies.

First, the nature of the "treatment"—the smoking ban and collateral programs—is far from clear in specific studies, so there may not be a common intervention to assess. Any form of causal analysis needs to be explicit about the details of the intervention and the fidelity with which it was implemented. In addition, some of the studies tested different "treatments" as part of their hypotheses: some looked simply at the effect of smoking bans, others looked more directly at changes in secondhand-smoke exposure.

Second, the population of interest varied from study to study in both explicit and implicit ways. Some looked at a population as a whole, others focused on smokers and nonsmokers separately. Population differences in responses to the interventions, such as changes in behavior, and differences in preexisting disease could exist. Those differences could be assessed and accounted for differently among studies, but many of the studies were silent on those issues; when they were not, they differed in how the issues are addressed.

Third, given the absence of randomization into treatment and nontreatment groups, the choice of comparison groups for assessing the effect of an intervention is problematic. The studies under review varied substantially in that regard. Some studies used historical controls, others used longitudinal statistical adjustments with such techniques as time-series analyses and stratification by demographic group. The problem with respect to estimating the magnitude of the overall effect is that the studies at hand did not adopt the same analytic strategy and did not make the ideal adjustments.

Fourth, the relative changes in the numbers of acute events appear to vary from study to study, and this poses problems in the examination of the heterogeneous responses to the interventions. There are two ways to try to deal with such heterogeneity: include possible confounding variables as part of the model to remove heterogeneity by adjustment, and consider adding an extra component of variation in the error term for heterogeneity to make the standard errors larger than they would have been if the results had been homogeneous. Several of the studies included adjustment variables to capture effects of demographic groups, seasonality, or both, but each made such adjustments differently. Small numbers of events, as observed in several of the studies, militate against elaborate statistical adjustments for demographic groups or considerations of seasonality, and the adjustments that several of the studies made appear far from optimal. That leaves open the question of whether studies should focus on individual-level rather than group-level assessments and, if so, how they should do that.

Finally, the studies varied widely in their measures of acute cardiovascular events and in the time until differences were observed. In some instances, investigators allowed the time to effect to be determined by the data; in others, they hypothesized different periods.

When all those and other factors are taken into account, no simple meta-analytic technique is adequate for assessing the magnitude of the effect of a smoking ban or of the effect of a reduction in exposure to secondhand smoke on acute cardiovascular events.

In summary, the studies all appear to have found substantial reductions in acute cardiovascular events after the implementation of smoking bans and in that sense were consistent, but separately and collectively they had statistical shortcomings. The committee concludes that the shortcomings do not negate the evidence of an association between smoking bans and the incidence of acute MI or, for the relevant studies, secondhand-smoke exposure and the incidence of acute MI. As a consequence of the variability and the limitations, however, it is difficult to use them to estimate the magnitude of the effect of smoking bans or secondhand-smoke exposure on the incidence of acute MI.

CONCLUSIONS

- The extent to which the studies assessed possible alternative causes of changes in hospitalizations—health-care availability, use of different cardiac medications, new diagnostic criteria, and a decrease in all hospital admissions during a period—should be considered, especially if before–after comparisons are being made in the absence of a comparison area. Given the multiple factors that could affect the rate of acute MIs, however, an assessment of secular trends is preferable.
- Results of studies that included self-reported assessments of exposure to secondhand smoke cannot necessarily be compared with results of other studies that did the same thing unless the survey instruments (such as interviews) were similar.
- All the studies are relevant and informative with respect to the questions posed to the committee, and overall they support an association between smoking bans and a decrease in acute cardiovascular events.
- The magnitude of the effect cannot be determined on the basis of the studies, because of variability among and uncertainties within them.
- In most of the studies, the portion of the effect attributable to decreased smoking by smokers as opposed to decreased exposure of nonsmokers to secondhand smoke cannot be determined.
- The studies support, to the extent that it was evaluated, an association between a reduction in secondhand smoke and a decrease in acute cardiovascular events. The strongest data on that association in nonsmokers come from
  - Analyses of only nonsmokers (Monroe, Indiana, and Scotland).
  - Analyses that showed decreases in secondhand smoke after implementation of smoking bans.
- At the population level, results of the key intervention studies reviewed by the committee are for the most part consistent with a decrease in risk as early as a month following reductions in secondhand-smoke exposure; however, given the variability in the

studies and the lack of data on the precise timing of interventions, the smoking-ban studies do not provide adequate information on the time it takes to see decreases in cardiovascular effects.
- The results of the studies are consistent with the findings of the pathophysiologic studies discussed in Chapter 3.

REFERENCES

Akbar-Khanzadeh, F., S. Milz, A. Ames, S. Spino, and C. Tex. 2004. Effectiveness of clean indoor air ordinances in controlling environmental tobacco smoke in restaurants. *Archives of Environmental Health* 59(12):677-685.

Alpert, H. R., C. M. Carpenter, M. J. Travers, and G. N. Connolly. 2007. Environmental and economic evaluation of the Massachusetts smoke-free workplace law. *Journal of Community Health* 32(4):269-281.

Anderson, R. N., A. M. Minino, D. L. Hoyert, and H. M. Rosenberg. 2001. Comparability of cause of death between *ICD-9* and *ICD-10*: Preliminary estimates. *National Vital Statistics Report* 49(2):1-32.

Barone-Adesi, F., L. Vizzini, F. Merletti, and L. Richiardi. 2006. Short-term effects of Italian smoking regulation on rates of hospital admission for acute myocardial infarction. *European Heart Journal* 27(20):2468-2472.

Bartecchi, C., R. N. Alsever, C. Nevin-Woods, W. M. Thomas, R. O. Estacio, B. B. Bartelson, and M. J. Krantz. 2006. Reduction in the incidence of acute myocardial infarction associated with a citywide smoking ordinance. *Circulation* 114(14):1490-1496.

CDC (Centers for Disease Control and Prevention). 2004. Indoor air quality in hospitality venues before and after implementation of a clean indoor air law—western New York, 2003. *MMWR—Morbidity & Mortality Weekly Report* 53(44):1038-1041.

———. 2007. Reduced secondhand smoke exposure after implementation of a comprehensive statewide smoking ban—New York, June 26, 2003–June 30, 2004. *MMWR—Morbidity & Mortality Weekly Report* 56(28):705-708.

———. 2009. Reduced hospitalizations for acute myocardial infarction after implementation of a smoke-free ordinance—city of Pueblo, Colorado, 2002–2006. *MMWR—Morbidity & Mortality Weekly Report* 57(51):1373-1377.

Cesaroni, G., F. Forastiere, N. Agabiti, P. Valente, P. Zuccaro, and C. A. Perucci. 2008. Effect of the Italian smoking ban on population rates of acute coronary events. *Circulation* 117(9):1183-1188.

Cirera Suarez, L., M. Rodriguez Barranco, E. Madrigal de Torres, J. Carillo Prieto, A. Hasiak Santo, R. Augusto Becker, A. Tobias Garcés, and N. Sánchez Carmen. 2006. [Correspondences from 10th to 9th revision of the International Classification of Diseases in the causes of death lists of the National Institute of Statistics and the Regional Health Authority of Murcia in Spain]. *Revista Española de Salud Pública* 80(2):157-175.

Dockery, D. W. 2009. Health effects of particulate air pollution. *Annals of Epidemiology* 19(4):257-263.

Ellingsen, D. G., G. Fladseth, H. L. Daae, M. Gjolstad, K. Kjaerheim, M. Skogstad, R. Olsen, S. Thorud, and P. Molander. 2006. Airborne exposure and biological monitoring of bar and restaurant workers before and after the introduction of a smoking ban. *Journal of Environmental Monitoring* 8(3):362-368.

French, B., and P. J. Heagerty. 2008. Analysis of longitudinal data to evaluate a policy change. *Statistics in Medicine* 27(24):5005-5025.

Gallus, S., P. Zuccaro, P. Colombo, G. Apolone, R. Pacifici, S. Garattini, and C. La Vecchia. 2006. Effects of new smoking regulations in Italy. *Annals of Oncology* 17(2):346-347.

Gevecker Graves, C., M. E. Ginevan, R. A. Jenkins, and R. G. Tardiff. 2000. Doses and lung burdens of environmental tobacco smoke constituents in nonsmoking workplaces. *Journal of Exposure Analysis and Environmental Epidemiology* 10(4):365-377.

Glantz, S. 2008. Meta-analysis of the effects of smokefree laws on acute myocardial infarction: An update. *Preventive Medicine* 47:452-453.

Goldacre, M. J., S. E. Roberts, and M. Griffith. 2003. Multiple-cause coding of death from myocardial infarction: Population-based study of trends in death certificate data. *Journal of Public Health Medicine* 25(1):69-71.

Gorini, G., A. Gasparrini, M. C. Fondelli, A. S. Costantini, F. Centrich, M. J. Lopez, M. Nebot, and E. Tamang. 2005. Environmental tobacco smoke (ETS) exposure in Florence hospitality venues before and after the smoking ban in Italy. *Journal of Occupational & Environmental Medicine* 47(12):1208-1210; author reply 1210.

Griffiths, C., A. Brock, and C. Rooney. 2004. The impact of introducing ICD-10 on trends in mortality from circulatory diseases in England and Wales. *Health Statistics Quarterly* 22:14-20.

Haw, S. J., and L. Gruer. 2007. Changes in exposure of adult non-smokers to secondhand smoke after implementation of smoke-free legislation in Scotland: National Cross Sectional survey. *BMJ* 335(7619):549.

HEI (Health Effects Institute) Accountability Working Group. 2003. *Assessing the health impact of air quality regulations: Concepts and methods for accountability research. Communication 11.* Boston, MA: Health Effects Institute.

HHS (U.S. Department of Health and Human Services). 2008. *HHS proposes adoption of ICD-10 code sets and updated electronic transaction standards. Press release.* (Accessed March 1, 2009, from http://www.hhs.gov/news/press/2008pres/08/20080815a.html.)

Juster, H. R., B. R. Loomis, T. M. Hinman, M. C. Farrelly, A. Hyland, U. E. Bauer, and G. S. Birkhead. 2007. Declines in hospital admissions for acute myocardial infarction in New York state after implementation of a comprehensive smoking ban. *American Journal of Public Health* 97(11):2035-2039.

Kado, N. Y., S. A. McCurdy, S. J. Tesluk, S. K. Hammond, D. P. Hsieh, J. Jones, and M. B. Schenker. 1991. Measuring personal exposure to airborne mutagens and nicotine in environmental tobacco smoke. *Mutation Research* 261(1):75-82.

Kavsak, P. A., A. R. MacRae, V. Lustig, R. Bhargava, R. Vandersluis, G. E. Palomaki, M. J. Yerna, and A. S. Jaffe. 2006. The impact of the ESC/ACC redefinition of myocardial infarction and new sensitive troponin assays on the frequency of acute myocardial infarction. *American Heart Journal* 152(1):118-125.

Khuder, S. A., S. Milz, T. Jordan, J. Price, K. Silvestri, and P. Butler. 2007. The impact of a smoking ban on hospital admissions for coronary heart disease. *Preventive Medicine* 45(1):3-8.

Kircher, T., J. Nelson, and H. Burdo. 1985. The autopsy as a measure of accuracy of the death certificate. *New England Journal of Medicine* 313(20):1263-1269.

Leaderer, B. P., and S. K. Hammond. 1991. Evaluation of vapor-phase nicotine and respirable suspended particle mass as markers for environmental tobacco smoke. *Environmental Science and Technology* 25(4):770-777.

Lemstra, M., C. Neudorf, and J. Opondo. 2008. Implications of a public smoking ban. *Canadian Journal of Public Health* 99(1):62-65.

Lightwood, J. M., and S. A. Glantz. 2009. Declines in acute myocardial infarction after smoke-free laws and individual risk attributable to secondhand smoke. *Circulation* 120:1373-1379.

Lofroth, G., and G. Lazaridis. 1986. Environmental tobacco smoke: Comparative characterization by mutagenicity assays of sidestream and mainstream cigarette smoke. *Environmental Mutagenesis* 8(5):693-704.

Luepker, R. V., F. S. Apple, R. H. Christenson, R. S. Crow, S. P. Fortmann, D. Goff, R. J. Goldberg, M. M. Hand, A. S. Jaffe, D. G. Julian, D. Levy, T. Manolio, S. Mendis, G. Mensah, A. Pajak, R. J. Prineas, K. S. Reddy, V. L. Roger, W. D. Rosamond, E. Shahar, A. R. Sharrett, P. Sorlie, and H. Tunstall-Pedoe. 2003. Case definitions for acute coronary heart disease in epidemiology and clinical research studies: A statement from the AHA Council on Epidemiology and Prevention; AHA Statistics Committee; World Heart Federation Council on Epidemiology and Prevention; the European Society of Cardiology Working Group on Epidemiology and Prevention; Centers for Disease Control and Prevention; and the National Heart, Lung, and Blood Institute. *Circulation* 108(20):2543-2549.

Mahonen, M., V. Salomaa, M. Brommels, A. Molarius, H. Miettinen, K. Pyorala, J. Tuomilehto, M. Arstila, E. Kaarsalo, M. Ketonen, K. Kuulasmaa, S. Lehto, H. Mustaniemi, M. Niemela, P. Palomaki, J. Torppa, and T. Vuorenmaa. 1997. The validity of hospital discharge register data on coronary heart disease in Finland. *European Journal of Epidemiology* 13(4):403-415.

Menzies, D., A. Nair, P. A. Williamson, S. Schembri, M. Z. H. Al-Khairalla, M. Barnes, T. C. Fardon, L. McFarlane, G. J. Magee, and B. J. Lipworth. 2006. Respiratory symptoms, pulmonary function, and markers of inflammation among bar workers before and after a legislative ban on smoking in public places. *JAMA* 296(14):1742-1748.

Nashelsky, M. B., and C. H. Lawrence. 2003. Accuracy of cause of death determination without forensic autopsy examination. *Am J Forensic Med Pathol* 24(4):313-319.

National Center for Health Statistics. 2009. *About the International Classification of Disease, Tenth Revision, Clinical Modification (ICD-10-CM).* (Accessed March 1, 2009, from http://www.cdc.gov/nchs/about/otheract/icd9/abticd10.htm.)

Pajunen, P., H. Koukkunen, M. Ketonen, T. Jerkkola, P. Immonen-Raiha, P. Karja-Koskenkari, M. Mahonen, M. Niemela, K. Kuulasmaa, P. Palomaki, J. Mustonen, A. Lehtonen, M. Arstila, T. Vuorenmaa, S. Lehto, H. Miettinen, J. Torppa, J. Tuomilehto, Y. A. Kesaniemi, K. Pyorala, and V. Salomaa. 2005. The validity of the Finnish Hospital Discharge Register and Causes of Death Register data on coronary heart disease. *European Journal of Cardiovascular Prevention & Rehabilitation* 12(2):132-137.

Pell, J. P., S. Haw, S. Cobbe, D. E. Newby, A. C. H. Pell, C. Fischbacher, A. McConnachie, S. Pringle, D. Murdoch, F. Dunn, K. Oldroyd, P. Macintyre, B. O'Rourke, and W. Borland. 2008. Smoke-free legislation and hospitalizations for acute coronary syndrome. *New England Journal of Medicine* 359(5):482-491.

Peng, R. D., H. H. Chang, M. L. Bell, A. McDermott, S. L. Zeger, J. M. Samet, and F. Dominici. 2008. Coarse particulate matter air pollution and hospital admissions for cardiovascular and respiratory diseases among medicare patients. *JAMA* 299(18):2172-2179.

Pladevall, M., D. C. Goff, M. Z. Nichaman, F. Chan, D. Ramsey, C. Ortiz, and D. R. Labarthe. 1996. An assessment of the validity of ICD code 410 to identify hospital admissions for myocardial infarction: The Corpus Christi Heart Project. *International Journal of Epidemiology* 25(5):948-952.

Ravakhah, K. 2006. Death certificates are not reliable: Revivification of the autopsy. *Southern Medical Journal* 99(7):729-733.

Richiardi, L., L. Vizzini, F. Merletti, and F. Barone-Adesi. 2009. Cardiovascular benefits of smoking regulations: The effect of decreased exposure to passive smoking. *Preventive Medicine* 48(2):167-172.

RTI (Research Triangle Institute) International. 2004. *First annual independent evaluation of New York's Tobacco Control Program: Final report.* Research Triangle Park, NC.

Rubin, D. B. 2008. For objective causal inference, design trumps analysis. *Annals of Applied Statistics* 2(3):808-840.

Sargent, R. P., R. M. Shepard, and S. A. Glantz. 2004. Reduced incidence of admissions for myocardial infarction associated with public smoking ban: Before and after study. *BMJ* 328(7446):977-980.

Semple, S., K. S. Creely, A. Naji, B. G. Miller, and J. G. Ayres. 2007a. Secondhand smoke levels in Scottish pubs: The effect of smoke-free legislation. *Tobacco Control* 16(2):127-132.

Semple, S., L. Maccalman, A. A. Naji, S. Dempsey, S. Hilton, B. G. Miller, and J. G. Ayres. 2007b. Bar workers' exposure to second-hand smoke: The effect of Scottish smoke-free legislation on occupational exposure. *Annals of Occupational Hygiene* 51(7):571-580.

Seo, D.-C., and M. R. Torabi. 2007. Reduced admissions for acute myocardial infarction associated with a public smoking ban: Matched controlled study. *Journal of Drug Education* 37(3):217-226.

Stranges, S., M. R. Bonner, F. Fucci, K. M. Cummings, J. L. Freudenheim, J. M. Dorn, P. Muti, G. A. Giovino, A. Hyland, and M. Trevisan. 2006. Lifetime cumulative exposure to secondhand smoke and risk of myocardial infarction in never smokers: Results from the western New York Health study, 1995-2001. *Archives of Internal Medicine* 166(18):1961-1967.

Teo, K. K., S. Ounpuu, S. Hawken, M. R. Pandey, V. Valentin, D. Hunt, R. Diaz, W. Rashed, R. Freeman, L. Jiang, X. Zhang, and S. Yusuf. 2006. Tobacco use and risk of myocardial infarction in 52 countries in the INTERHEART study: A case-control study. *Lancet* 368(9536):647-658.

Valente, P., F. Forastiere, A. Bacosi, G. Cattani, S. Di Carlo, M. Ferri, I. Figa-Talamanca, A. Marconi, L. Paoletti, C. Perucci, and P. Zuccaro. 2007. Exposure to fine and ultrafine particles from secondhand smoke in public places before and after the smoking ban, Italy 2005. *Tobacco Control* 16(5):312-317.

Vasselli, S., P. Papini, D. Gaelone, L. Spizzichino, E. De Campora, R. Gnavi, C. Saitto, N. Binkin, and G. Laurendi. 2008. Reduction incidence of myocardial infarction associated with a national legislative ban on smoking. *Minerva Cardioangiologica* 56(2):197-203.

WHO (World Health Organization). 2009. International Classification of Diseases *(ICD)* (Accessed March 1, 2009, from http://www.who.int/classifications/icd/en/.)

8

Conclusions and Recommendations

In this report, the committee has examined three relationships in response to its charge (see Box 8-1 for specific questions):

- The association between secondhand-smoke exposure and cardiovascular disease, especially coronary heart disease and not stroke (Question 1).
- The association between secondhand-smoke exposure and acute coronary events (Questions 2, 3, and 5).
- The association between smoking bans and acute coronary events (Questions 4, 5, 6, 7, and 8).

This chapter summarizes the committee's review of information relevant to those relationships; presents its findings, conclusions, and recommendations on the basis of the weight of evidence; and presents its responses to the specific questions that it was asked in its task.

SUMMARY OF REPORT

Exposure Assessment

To determine the effect of changes in exposure to secondhand smoke it is necessary to quantify changes in epidemiologic studies. Airborne measures and biomarkers of exposure to secondhand smoke are available; they are complementary and provide different information (see Chapter 2). Biomarkers (such as cotinine, the major proximate metabolite of nicotine) in-

---

BOX 8-1
Specific Questions to the Committee

The Centers for Disease Control and Prevention requested that the IOM convene an expert committee to assess the state of the science on the relationship between secondhand smoke exposure and acute coronary events. Specifically, the committee was to review available scientific literature on secondhand smoke exposure (including short-term exposure) and acute coronary events, and produce a report characterizing the state of the science on the topic, with emphasis on the evidence for causality and knowledge gaps that future research should address.

In conducting its work the committee was to address the following questions:

1. What is the current scientific consensus on the relationship between exposure to secondhand smoke and cardiovascular disease? What is the pathophysiology? What is the strength of the relationship?
2. Is there sufficient evidence to support the plausibility of a causal relation between secondhand smoke exposure and acute coronary events such as acute myocardial infarction and unstable angina? If yes, what is the pathophysiology? And what is the strength of the relationship?
3. Is it biologically plausible that a relatively brief (e.g., under 1 hour) secondhand smoke exposure incident could precipitate an acute

---

tegrate all sources of exposure and inhalation rates, but cannot identify the place where secondhand-smoke exposure occurred and, because of a short half-life they reflect only recent exposures. Airborne measures of exposure can demonstrate the contribution of different sources or venues of exposure and can be used to measure changes in secondhand-smoke concentrations at individual venues, but they do not reflect the true dose. Airborne concentration of nicotine is a specific tracer for secondhand smoke. Particulate matter (PM) can also be used as an indicator of secondhand-smoke exposure, but because there are other sources of PM it is a less specific tracer than nicotine. The concentration of cotinine in serum, saliva, or urine is a specific indicator of integrated exposure to secondhand smoke.

Although in most of the smoking-ban studies the magnitude, frequency, and duration of exposures that occurred before a ban are not known, monitoring studies demonstrate that exposure to secondhand smoke is dramatically reduced in places that are covered by bans. Airborne nicotine

coronary event? If yes, what is known or suspected about how this risk may vary based upon absence or presence (and extent) of preexisting coronary artery disease?

4. What is the strength of the evidence for a causal relationship between indoor smoking bans and decreased risk of acute myocardial infarction?

5. What is a reasonable latency period between a decrease in secondhand smoke exposure and a decrease in risk of an acute myocardial infarction for an individual? What is a reasonable latency period between a decrease in population secondhand smoke exposure and a measurable decrease in acute myocardial infarction rates for a population?

6. What are the strengths and weaknesses of published population-based studies on the risk of acute myocardial infarction following the institution of comprehensive indoor smoking bans? In light of published studies' strengths and weaknesses, how much confidence is warranted in reported effect size estimates?

7. What factors would be expected to influence the effect size? For example, population age distribution, baseline level of secondhand smoke protection among nonsmokers, and level of secondhand smoke protection provided by the smoke-free law.

8. What are the most critical research gaps that should be addressed to improve our understanding of the impact of indoor air policies on acute coronary events? What studies should be performed to address these gaps?

and PM concentrations in regulated venues such as workplaces, bars, and restaurants decreased by more than 80% in most studies; serum, salivary, or urinary cotinine concentrations decreased by 50% or more in most studies, probably reflecting continuing exposures in unregulated venues (for example, in homes and cars).

Pathophysiology

The pathophysiology of the induction of cardiovascular disease by cigarette-smoking and secondhand-smoke exposure is complex and undoubtedly involves multiple agents. Many chemicals in secondhand smoke have been shown to exert cardiovascular toxicity (see Table 3-1), and both acute and chronic effects of these chemicals have been identified. Experimental studies in humans, animals, and cell cultures have demonstrated effects of secondhand smoke, its components (such as PM, acrolein, polycyclic aromatic hydrocarbons [PAHs], and metals), or both on the cardiovascular system (see Figure 3-1 for summary). Those studies have yielded sufficient evidence to support an inference that acute exposure to secondhand smoke induces endothelial dysfunction, increases thrombosis, causes inflammation, and potentially affects plaque stability adversely. Those effects appear at concentrations expected to be experienced by people exposed to second-hand smoke.

Data from animal studies also support a dose–response relationship between secondhand-smoke exposure and cardiovascular effects (see Chapter 3). The relationship is consistent with the understanding of the pathophysiology of coronary heart disease and the effects of secondhand smoke on humans, including chamber studies. The association comports with known associations between PM, a major constituent of secondhand smoke, and coronary heart disease.

Overall, the pathophysiologic data indicate that it is biologically plausible for secondhand-smoke exposure to have cardiovascular effects, such as effects that lead to cardiovascular disease and acute myocardial infarction (MI). The exact mechanisms by which such effects occur, however, remain to be elucidated.

Smoking-Ban Background

Characteristics of smoking bans can heavily influence their consequences. Interpretation of the results of epidemiologic studies that involve smoking bans must account for information on the bans and their enforcement.

Secondhand smoke should have been measured before and after implementation of a ban, and locations with and without bans should have been compared. Studies that include self-reported assessments of exposure to secondhand smoke cannot necessarily be compared with each other unless the survey instruments (such as interviews) were similar.

The comparability of the time and length of followup of the studies should be assessed. For example, the impact of a ban in one area may differ from the impact of a ban in another solely because the observation times were different and other activities may have occurred during the same periods. In comparing studies, it may be impossible to separate contextual factors associated with ban legislation—such as public comment periods, information announcing the ban, and notices about the impending changes—from the impact of the ban itself. The committee therefore included such contextual factors in drawing conclusions about the effects of a ban.

Interpretation needs to consider the timeframes in the epidemiologic evidence, for example, the time from onset of a smoking ban to the measurement of incidence of a disease, the timing and nature of enforcement, and the time until changes in cardiovascular-event rates were observed in people who had various baseline risks. Interpretation should account for the extent to which studies assessed possible alternative causes of decreases in hospitalizations for coronary events, including changes in health-care availability and in the standard of practice in cardiac care, such as new diagnostic criteria for acute MI during the period of study. The latter is especially important in making before–after comparisons in the absence of a comparison geographic area in which no ban has been implemented.

When designing and analyzing future studies, researchers should examine the time between the implementation of a smoking ban and changes in rates of hospital admission or cardiac death. Future studies could evaluate whether decreases in admissions are transitory, sustained, or increasing, and ideally they would include information on individual subjects, including prior history of cardiac disease, to answer the questions posed to the committee.

Epidemiologic Studies

Cardiovascular disease is a major public-health concern. The results of dozens of epidemiologic studies of both case–control and cohort design carried out in multiple populations consistently indicate about a 25–30% increase in risk of coronary heart disease from exposure to secondhand smoke (see Chapter 4). Epidemiologic studies using serum cotinine concentration as a biomarker of overall exposure to secondhand smoke indicated that the relative risk (RR) of coronary heart disease associated with secondhand smoke is even greater than those estimates. The excess risk is unlikely to be explained by misclassification bias, uncontrolled-for confounding effects, or publication bias. Although few studies have addressed the risk of coronary heart disease posed by secondhand-smoke exposure in the workplace, there is no biologically plausible reason to suppose that the effect of secondhand-smoke exposure at work or in a public building differs from the effect of exposure in the home environment. Epidemiologic studies demonstrate a dose–response relationship between chronic secondhand-smoke exposure as assessed by self-reports of exposure (He et al., 1999) and as assessed by biomarkers (cotinine) and long-term risk of coronary heart disease (Whincup et al., 2004). Dose–response curves show a steep initial rise in risk when going from negligible to low exposure followed by a gradual increase with increasing exposure.

The INTERHEART study, a large case–control study of cases of first acute MI, showed that exposure to secondhand smoke increased the risk of nonfatal acute MI in a graded manner (Teo et al., 2006).

Eleven key epidemiologic studies evaluated the effects of eight smoking bans on the incidence of acute coronary events (see Table 8-1 and Chapter 6). The results of those studies show remarkable consistency: all showed decreases in the rate of acute MIs after the implementation of smoking bans (Barone-Adesi et al., 2006; Bartecchi et al., 2006; CDC, 2009; Cesaroni et al., 2008; Juster et al., 2007; Khuder et al., 2007; Lemstra et al., 2008; Pell et al., 2008; Sargent et al., 2004; Seo and Torabi, 2007; Vasselli et al., 2008). Two of the studies (Pell et al., 2008; Seo and Torabi, 2007) examined rates of hospitalization for acute coronary events after the implementation of smoking bans and provided direct evidence of the relationship of secondhand-smoke exposure to acute coronary events by presenting results in nonsmokers.

The decreases in acute MIs in the 11 studies ranged from about 6 to 47%, depending on characteristics of the study, including the method of statistical analysis. The consistency in the direction of change gave the committee confidence that smoking bans result in a decrease in the rate of acute MI. The studies took advantage of bans as "natural experiments" to look at questions about the effects of bans, and indirectly of a decrease in secondhand-smoke exposure, on the incidence of acute cardiac events. As discussed in *Assessing the Health Impact of Air Quality Regulations: Concepts and Methods for Accountability Research* (HEI Accountability Working Group, 2003) in the context of air-pollution regulations, studies of interventions constitute a more definitive approach than other epidemiologic studies to determining whether regulations result in health benefits. All the studies are relevant and informative with respect to the questions posed to the committee, and overall they support an association between smoking bans and a decrease in acute cardiovascular events. The studies have inherent limitations related to their nature, but they directly evaluated the effects of an intervention (a smoking ban, including any concomitant activities) on a health outcome of interest (acute coronary events).

The committee could not determine the magnitude of effect with any reasonable degree of certainty on the basis of those studies. The variability in study design, implementation, and analysis was so large that the committee concluded that it could not conduct a meta-analysis or combine the information from the studies to calculate a point estimate of the effect. In particular, the committee was unable to determine the overall portion of the effect attributable to decreased smoking by smokers as opposed to decreased exposure of nonsmokers to secondhand smoke because of a lack of information on smoking status in nine of the studies (Barone-Adesi et al., 2006; Bartecchi et al., 2006; CDC, 2009; Cesaroni et al., 2008; Juster et al., 2007; Khuder et al., 2007; Lemstra et al., 2008; Sargent et al., 2004; Seo and Torabi, 2007; Vasselli et al., 2008). The results of the studies are consistent with the findings of the pathophysiologic studies discussed in Chapter 3 and the data on PM discussed in Chapters 3 and 7. At the population level, results of the key intervention studies reviewed by the committee are for the most part consistent with a decrease in risk as early as a month following reductions in secondhand-smoke exposure; however, given the variability in the studies and the lack of data on the precise timing of interventions, the smoking-ban studies do not provide adequate information on the time it takes to see decreases in acute MIs.

Plausibility of Effect

The committee considered both the biologic plausibility of a causal relationship between a decrease in secondhand-smoke exposure and a decrease in the incidence of acute MI and the plausibility of the magnitude of the effect seen in the key epidemiologic studies after implementation of smoking bans.

The experimental data reviewed in Chapter 3 demonstrate that several components of secondhand smoke, as well as secondhand smoke itself, exert substantial cardiovascular toxicity. The toxic effects include the induction of endothelial dysfunction, an increase in thrombosis, increased inflammation, and possible reductions in plaque stability. The data provide evidence that it is biologically plausible for secondhand smoke to be a potential causative trigger of acute coronary events. The risk of acute coronary events is likely to be increased if a person has preexisting heart disease. The association comports with findings on air-pollution components, such as diesel exhaust (Mills et al., 2007) and PM (Bhatnagar, 2006).

As a "reality check" on the potential effects of changes in secondhand-smoke exposure, the committee estimated the decrease in risk of cardiovascular disease and specifically heart failure that would be expected on the basis of the risk effects of changes in airborne PM concentrations after implementation of smoking bans seen in the PM literature. The PM in cigarette smoke is not identical with that in air pollution, and the committee did not attempt to estimate the risk attributable to secondhand-smoke exposure through the PM risk estimates but rather found this a useful exercise to see whether the decreases seen in the epidemiologic literature are reasonable, given data on other air pollutants that have some common characteristics. The committee's estimates on the basis of the PM literature support the possibility that changes in secondhand-smoke exposure after implementation of a smoking ban can have a substantial effect on hospital admissions for heart failure and cardiovascular disease.

SUMMARY OF OVERALL WEIGHT OF EVIDENCE

The committee examined three relationships—of secondhand-smoke exposure and cardiovascular disease, of secondhand-smoke exposure and

TABLE 8-1 Summary of Key Studies (Studies Listed by Smoking-Ban Region in Order of Publication)

Publication (Region)	Study Design and Duration
Helena, Montana	
Sargent et al., 2004 (Helena, Montana)	Retrospective based on hospital records; 6 months of ban, 11 months after ban compared with same months of 5 years before ban
Italy	
Vasselli et al., 2008 (four regions in Italy: Piedmont, Friuli–Venezia–Giulia, Latium, Campania)	Retrospective based on hospital discharge registry; study period January 10–March 10, 2001–2005; compared 2 months after ban with same 2 months of 4 years before ban
Barone-Adesi et al., 2006 (Piedmont region, northern Italy)	Retrospective based on records from regional hospital discharge registry; 5 months before ban studied, ending 6 months before implementation; 6 months after ban studied
Cesaroni et al., 2008 (Rome, Italy)	Retrospective based on hospital discharge registry, death registry; January 1, 2000–December 31, 2005; follow-up just under 12 months after ban
Pueblo, Colorado	
CDC, 2009 (Pueblo, Colorado)	Retrospective based on hospital admission data; duration 1.5 years before, 1.5 and 3 years after ban
Bartecchi et al., 2006 (Pueblo, Colorada)	Same as CDC (2009) but only after 1.5 years of followup
Monroe County, Indiana	
Seo and Torabi, 2007 (Monroe County, Indiana)	Retrospective based on records; study period August 1, 2001–May 31, 2005, that is, 22 months before and 22 months after ban's enforcement
Bowling Green, Ohio	
Khuder et al., 2007 (Bowling Green, Ohio)	Retrospective based on hospital discharge records in 1999–2005; assessment from October 2002 to 39 months after ban went into effect (March 2002)

Ban Characteristics	Decrease in Admission Rates
Legislation enacted to require smoke-free workplaces, public places, including restaurants, bars; suspended after about 6 months Smoking banned in restaurants, bars, other workplaces	40% decrease in average monthly admissions (from 40 to 24; decrease of 16 cases, 95% CI)
Ban on smoking in all indoor public places, including offices, retail shops, cafes, bars, restaurants, discotheques in Italy; provision for smoking rooms Ban on smoking in all indoor public places, including offices, retail shops, cafes, bars, restaurants, discotheques in Italy; provision for smoking rooms Ban on smoking in all indoor public places, including offices, retail shops, cafes, bars, restaurants, discotheques in Italy; provision for smoking rooms	6.4% decrease from previous year 13.1% decrease (estimated) from expected on basis of linear regression (RR, 0.6; 95% CI, 0.83–0.92) 11% decrease in people under 60 years old (RR, 0.89; 95% CI, 0.81–0.98) 11% decrease in people 35–64 years old (RR, 0.89; 95% CI, 0.85–0.93) 8% decrease in people 65–74 years old (RR, 0.92; 95% CI, 0.88–0.97)
Ban prohibiting smoking in workplaces, all public buildings—including restaurants, bars, bowling alleys, other business establishments—in city limits Ban prohibiting smoking in workplaces, all public buildings—including restaurants, bars, bowling alleys, other business establishments—in city limits	41% decrease (RR, 0.59; 95% CI, 0.49–0.70) 27% decrease (RR, 0.73; 95% CI, 0.63–0.85)
Ban in all restaurants, retail stores, workplaces; extended to previously exempt bars and clubs January 1, 2005	70% decrease (from 17 to 5; decrease of 12 cases, 95% CI, 2.81–21.19)
Ban in public places except bars, restaurants with bars if bar is isolated with separate smoking area; bars and bowling alleys could allow smoking at owners' discretion	39% decrease (95% CI, 33–45%) in 2002 (includes 2 months without ordinance) for 9–21 months of followup 47% decrease (95% CI, 41–55%) for 34–39 months of followup

Continued

TABLE 8-1 Continued

Publication (Region)	Study Design and Duration
New York State Juster et al., 2007 (New York state)	Retrospective based on hospital discharge records; estimates of admissions calculated statistically; data for January 1995–December 2004 (17 months after statewide ban)
Saskatoon, Canada Lemstra et al., 2008 (Saskatoon, Canada)	Retrospective based on hospital discharge records; compared first full year after ban (July 1, 2004–June 30, 2005) with previous 4 years (July 1, 2000–June 30, 2004)
Scotland Pell et al., 2008 (Scotland)	Prospective study of acute coronary syndrome; 10 months before (June 2005–March 2006) and follow-up 10 months after (June 2006–March 2007) ban

Ban Characteristics	Decrease in Admission Rates
New York's Clean Indoor Air Act is 100% statewide ban on smoking in all workplaces—including restaurants, bars, gaming establishments—with limited exceptions Statewide smoking restrictions (limiting or prohibiting smoking in some public places, such as schools, hospitals, public buildings, retail stores) had been implemented in 1989 Previously, various levels of smoking bans implemented at city or county level in some parts of New York state, including ban in workplaces—including restaurants, bars—in New York City State law does not preempt passage of local laws	8% (estimated) fewer admissions in 2004 than expected with prior existing local smoking bans 19% (estimated) fewer admissions in 2004 than expected if no prior smoking bans had been in effect
Smoking ban implemented in city of Saskatoon prohibiting smoking in any enclosed public space that is open to public or to which public is customarily admitted or invited; smoking also prohibited in outdoor seating areas of restaurants, licensed premises Previously, smoking had been prohibited in government buildings As of January 1, 2005, 100% smoke-free law in all public places, workplaces, including restaurants, bars, bingo halls, bowling alleys, casinos; local municipalities have right to enact smoke-free air regulations	13% decrease (rate ratio, 0.87; 95% CI, 0.84–0.90)
Smoking prohibited in all enclosed public places, workplaces throughout Scotland, including bars, pubs, restaurants, cafes; exceptions included residential accommodations, designated rooms in hotels, care homes, hospices, psychiatric units	17% decrease (95% CI, 16–18%) after implementation of smoking ban

acute coronary events, and of smoking bans and acute coronary events. The committee used the criteria of causation described in *Smoking and Health: Report of the Advisory Committee of the Surgeon General of the Public Health Service* (U.S. Public Health Service, 1964) in drawing conclusions regarding those relationships. The criteria are often referred to as the Bradford Hill criteria because they were, as stated by Hamill (1997), "later expanded and refined by A. B. Hill" (Hill, 1965). Table 8-2 summarizes the available evidence on secondhand-smoke exposure and coronary events in terms of the Bradford Hill criteria.

Secondhand-Smoke Exposure and Cardiovascular Disease

The results of both case–control and cohort studies carried out in multiple populations consistently indicate exposure to secondhand smoke causes about a 25–30% increase in the risk of coronary heart disease; results of some studies indicate a dose–response relationship. Data from animal studies support the dose–response relationship (see Chapter 3). Data from experimental studies of animals and cells and from intentional human-dosing studies indicate that a relationship between secondhand-smoke exposure and coronary heart disease is biologically plausible and consistent with understanding of the pathophysiology of coronary heart disease.

Taking all that evidence together, the committee concurs with the conclusions in the 2006 surgeon general's report (HHS, 2006) that "the evidence is sufficient to infer a causal relationship between exposure to secondhand smoke and increased risks of coronary heart disease morbidity and mortality among both men and women." Although the committee found strong and consistent evidence of the existence of a positive association between chronic exposure to secondhand smoke and coronary heart disease, determining the magnitude of the risk (the number of cases that are attributable to secondhand-smoke exposure) proved challenging, and the committee has not done it.

Secondhand-Smoke Exposure and Acute Coronary Events

Two of the epidemiologic studies reviewed by the committee that examine rates of hospitalization for acute coronary events after implementation of smoking bans provide direct evidence related to secondhand smoke exposures. The studies either reported events in nonsmokers only (Monroe, Indiana) (Seo and Torabi, 2007) or analyzed nonsmokers and smokers separately on the basis of serum cotinine concentration (Scotland) (Pell et al., 2008). Both studies showed reductions in the RR of acute coronary events in nonsmokers when secondhand-smoke exposure was decreased after implementation of the bans; this indicates an association between a decrease in exposure to secondhand smoke and a decrease in risk of acute coronary events. Because of differences between and limitations of the two studies (such as in population, population size, and analysis), they do not provide strong sufficient evidence to determine the magnitude of the decrease in RR.

The effect seen after implementation of smoking bans is consistent with data from the INTERHEART study, a case–control study of 15,152 cases of first acute MI in 262 centers in 52 countries (Teo et al., 2006). Increased exposure to secondhand smoke increased the risk of nonfatal acute MI in a graded manner, with adjusted odds ratios of 1.24 (95% confidence interval [CI], 1.17–1.32) and 1.62 (95% CI, 1.45–1.81) in the least exposed people (1–7 hours of exposure per week) and the most exposed (at least 22 hours of exposure per week), respectively. In contrast, a study using data from the Western New York Health Study collected from 1995 to 2001 found that secondhand smoke was not significantly associated with higher risk of MI (Stranges et al., 2007). That study, however, looked at lifetime cumulative exposure to secondhand smoke, a different exposure metric from that in the other studies and one that does not take into account how recent the exposure is.

The other key epidemiologic studies that looked at smoking bans provide indirect evidence of an association between secondhand-smoke exposure and acute coronary events (Barone-Adesi et al., 2006; Bartecchi et al., 2006; CDC, 2009; Cesaroni et al., 2008; Juster et al., 2007; Khuder et al., 2007; Lemstra et al., 2008; Sargent et al., 2004; Vasselli et al., 2008). Although it is not possible to separate the effect of smoking bans in reducing exposure to secondhand smoke and their effect in reducing active smoking in those studies, because they did not report individual smoking status or secondhand-smoke exposure concentrations, monitoring studies of airborne tracers[1] and biomarkers[2] of exposure to secondhand smoke have demonstrated that exposure to secondhand smoke is dramatically reduced after implementation of smoking bans. Those studies therefore provide indirect evidence that at least part of the decrease in acute coronary events seen after implementation of smoking bans could be mediated by a decrease in exposure to secondhand smoke. It is not possible to determine the differential magnitude of the effect that is attributable to changes in nonsmokers and smokers.

Experimental data show that an association between secondhand-

---

[1] Airborne measures of exposure, such as the unique tracer nicotine or the less specific tracer PM, can demonstrate the contribution of different sources or venues of an exposure but do not reflect true dose.

[2] Biomarkers of exposure to tobacco smoke, such as serum or salivary cotinine concentrations, integrate all sources of exposure and inhalation rates but, because of a short half-life, reflect only recent exposures.

TABLE 8-2 Evaluation of Available Data in Terms of Bradford-Hill Criteria

Bradford-Hill Criterion	Secondhand-Smoke Exposure and Cardiovascular Disease	Secondhand-Smoke Exposure and Acute Coronary Events	Smoking Bans and Acute Coronary Events
Strength of association[a]	Weak	Weak	Weak
Consistency	Yes	Yes	Yes, all published studies of smoking bans and acute coronary events have shown decrease in acute coronary events; however, bans are not identical interventions
Specificity	No, because there are many factors that contribute to cardiovascular disease. many effects of secondhand-smoke exposure	No, because there are many factors that contribute to cardiovascular disease, many effects of secondhand-smoke exposure	To some extent; some studies may include effects on smoking cessation
Temporality	Yes	Yes	Yes
Biologic gradient (dose–response relationship)	Yes. Where evaluated, epidemiologic studies show dose–response relationship for chronic exposure, probably associated with acute doses as well; animal studies show dose–response relationship	Data from INTERHEART study (Teo et al., 2006) suggest nonlinear dose–response relationship	Smoking bans are either present or absent, so gradients are not always relevant; although information on exposure levels before and after implementation of ban could provide some information relevant to biologic gradient, available information is inadequate

Biologic plausibility or coherence	Yes, effects are consistent with current understanding of pathophysiology of cardiovascular disease and effects of secondhand-smoke exposure in humans, including that in chamber studies	Yes, based on experimental data showing changes that might be expected to precipitate such events	Yes, in that secondhand-smoke exposure is associated with cardiovascular disease. Evidence indicates that smoking bans decrease secondhand-smoke exposure
Experimental evidence	Supported by in vitro and in vivo evidence	Yes, for pathophysiologic changes related to acute coronary events	Not directly relevant to ban
Analogy	Association comports with what is known about particulate-matter pollution and cardiovascular disease	Association comports with what is known about particulate-matter pollution and acute coronary events	Association comports with what is known about particulate-matter pollution, secondhand-smoke exposure, and coronary heart disease

[a] Strength of association is categorized as "weak" because effect estimates are generally small, are variable, or both.

smoke exposure and acute coronary events is biologically plausible (see Chapter 3). Experimental studies in humans, animals, and cell cultures have demonstrated short-term effects of secondhand smoke as a complex mixture or its components individually (such as oxidants, PM, acrolein, PAHs, benzene, and metals) on the cardiovascular system. There is sufficient evidence from such studies to infer that acute exposure to secondhand smoke at concentrations relevant to population exposures induces endothelial dysfunction, increases inflammation, increases thrombosis, and potentially adversely affects plaque stability. Those effects occur at magnitudes relevant to the pathogenesis of acute coronary events. Furthermore, indirect evidence obtained from studies of ambient PM supports the notion that exposure to PM present in secondhand smoke could trigger acute coronary events or induce arrhythmogenesis in a person with a vulnerable myocardium.

Taking all that evidence together, the committee concludes that there is sufficient evidence of a causal relationship between a decrease in secondhand-smoke exposure and a decrease in the risk of acute MI. Given the variability among studies and their limitations, the committee did not provide a quantitative estimate of the magnitude of the effect.

Smoking Bans and Acute Coronary Events

Nine key studies looked at the overall effect of smoking bans on the incidence of acute coronary events in the overall populations—smokers and nonsmokers—studied (Barone-Adesi et al., 2006; Bartecchi et al., 2006; CDC, 2009; Cesaroni et al., 2008; Juster et al., 2007; Khuder et al., 2007; Lemstra et al., 2008; Sargent et al., 2004; Vasselli et al., 2008). Those studies consistently show a decrease in acute MIs after implementation of smoking bans. The combination of experimental data on secondhand-smoke effects discussed above and exposure data that indicate that secondhand-smoke concentrations decrease substantially after implementation of a smoking ban provides evidence that it is biologically plausible for smoking bans to decrease the rate of acute MIs. The committee concludes that there is an association between smoking bans and a reduction in acute coronary events and, given the temporality and biologic plausibility of the effect, that the evidence is consistent with a causal relationship. Although all the studies demonstrated a positive effect of bans in reducing acute MIs, differences among the studies, including the components of the bans and other interventions that promote smoke-free environments that took place during the bans, limited the committee's confidence in estimating the overall magnitude of the effect. There is little information on how long it would take for such an effect to be seen inasmuch as the studies have not evaluated periods shorter than a month.

DATA GAPS AND RESEARCH RECOMMENDATIONS

Studies of the effect of indoor smoking bans and secondhand-smoke exposure on acute coronary events should be designed to examine the time between an intervention and changes in the effect and to measure the magnitude of the effect. No time to effect can be postulated for individuals on the basis of the available data, and evaluation of population-based effectiveness of a smoking ban depends on societal actions that implement and enforce the ban and on actions that include smoke reduction in homes, cars, and elsewhere. The decrease in secondhand-smoke exposure does not necessarily occur suddenly—it might decline gradually or by steps. In a likely scenario, once a ban is put into place and enforced, a sharp drop in secondhand-smoke exposure might be seen immediately and followed by a slower decrease in exposure as the population becomes more educated about the health consequences of secondhand smoke and exposure becomes less socially acceptable. Future studies that examine the time from initiation of a ban to observation of an effect and that include followup after initiation of enforcement, taking the social aspects into account, would provide better information on how long it takes to see an effect of a ban. Statistical models should clearly articulate a set of assumptions and include sensitivity analyses. Studies that examine whether decreases in hospital admissions for acute coronary events are transitory or sustained would also be informative.

Many factors are likely to influence the effect of a smoking ban on the incidence and prevalence of acute coronary events in a population. They include age, sex, diet, background risk factors and environmental factors for cardiovascular disease, prevalence of smokers in the community, the underlying rate of heart disease in the community (for example, the rate in Italy versus the United States), and the social environment. Future studies should include direct observations on individuals—including their history of cardiac disease, exposure to other environmental agents, and other risk factors for cardiac events—to assess the impact of those factors on study results. Assessment of smoking status is also needed to distinguish between the effects of secondhand smoke in nonsmokers and the effects of a ban that decreases cigarette consumption or promotes smoking cessation in smokers.

Few constituents of secondhand smoke have been adequately studied for cardiotoxicity. Future research should examine the cardiotoxicity of environmental chemicals, including those in secondhand smoke, to define cardiovascular toxicity end points and establish consistent definitions and measurement standards for cardiotoxicity of environmental contaminants. Specifically, information is lacking on the cardiotoxicity of highly reactive smoke constituents, such as acrolein and other oxidants; on techniques for quantitating those reactive components; and on the toxicity of low concentrations of benzo[*a*]pyrene, of PAHs other than benzo[a]pyrene, and of mixtures of tobacco-smoke toxicants.

Many questions remain with respect to the pathogenesis of cardiovascular disease and acute coronary events and how secondhand-smoke constituents perturb the pathophysiologic mechanisms and result in disease and death. For example, a better understanding of the factors that promote plaque rupture and how they are influenced by tobacco smoke and PM would provide insight into the mechanisms underlying the cardiovascular effects of secondhand smoke and might lead to better methods of detecting preclinical disease and preventing events.

The committee found only sparse data on the prevalence and incidence of cardiovascular disease and acute coronary events at the national level in general compared with other health end points for which there are central data registries and surveillance of all events, such as the Surveillance, Epidemiology, and End Results (SEER) Program for cancer. Although there are national databases that include acute MI patients—such as the National Registry of Myocardial Infarction (Morrow et al., 2001; Rogers et al., 1994), the Health Care Financing Administration database, and the Cooperative Cardiovascular Project (Ellerbeck et al., 1995)—and the Centers for Disease Control and Prevention's annual National Hospital Discharge Survey and National Health Interview Survey provide some information on cardiovascular end points, these are not comprehensive or inclusive with respect to hospital participation, patient inclusion, or data capture. A national database that captures all cardiovascular end points would facilitate future epidemiologic studies by allowing the tracking of trends and identification of high-risk populations at a more granular level.

A large prospective cohort study could be very helpful in more accurately estimating the magnitude of the risk of cardiovascular disease and acute coronary events posed by secondhand-smoke exposure. It could be a new study specifically designed to assess effects of secondhand smoke or, as was done with the INTERHEART study, take advantage of existing studies—such as the Framingham Heart Study, the Multi-Ethnic Study of Atherosclerosis, the American Cancer Society's Cancer Prevention Study-3, the European Prospective Investigation into Cancer and Nutrition study, and the Jackson Heart Study—provided that they have adequate information on individual smoking status and secondhand-smoke exposure (or the ability to measure it, for example, in adequate blood samples). If properly designed, such a study could identify subpopulations at highest risk for acute coronary events from secondhand-smoke exposure in relation to such characteristics as age and sex, and concomitant risk factors, such as obesity.

COMMITTEE RESPONSES TO SPECIFIC QUESTIONS

The committee was tasked with responding to eight specific questions. The questions and the committee's responses are presented below.

1. *What is the current scientific consensus on the relationship between exposure to secondhand smoke and cardiovascular disease? What is the pathophysiology? What is the strength of the relationship?*

On the basis of the available studies of chronic exposure to secondhand smoke and cardiovascular disease, the committee concludes that there is scientific consensus that there is a causal relationship between secondhand-smoke exposure and cardiovascular disease. The results of a number of meta-analyses of the epidemiologic studies showed increases of 25–30% in the risk of cardiovascular disease caused by various exposures. The studies include some that use serum cotinine concentration as a biomarker of exposure and show a dose–response relationship. The pathophysiologic data are consistent with that relationship, as are the data from studies of air pollution and PM. The data in support of the relationship are consistent, but the committee could not calculate a point estimate of the magnitude of the effect (that is, the effect size) given the variable strength of the relationship, differences among studies, poor assessment of secondhand-smoke exposure, and variation in concomitant underlying risk factors.

2. *Is there sufficient evidence to support the plausibility of a causal relation between secondhand smoke exposure and acute coronary events such as acute myocardial infarction and unstable angina? If yes, what is the pathophysiology? And what is the strength of the relationship?*

The evidence reviewed by the committee is consistent with a causal relationship between secondhand-smoke exposure and acute coronary events, such as acute MI. It is unknown whether acute exposure, chronic exposure, or a combination of the two underlies the occurrence of acute coronary events, inasmuch as the duration or pattern of exposure in individuals is not known. The evidence includes the results of two key studies that have information on individual smoking status and that showed decreases in risks of acute coronary events in nonsmokers after implementation of a smoking ban. Those studies are supported by information from other smoking-ban studies (although these do not have information on individual smoking status, other exposure-assessment studies have demonstrated that secondhand-smoke exposure decreases after implementation of a smoking ban) and by the large body of literature on PM, especially $PM_{2.5}$, a constituent of secondhand smoke. The evidence is not yet comprehensive enough to determine a detailed mode of action for the relationship between secondhand-smoke exposure and a variety of intervening and preexisting conditions in predisposing to cardiac events. However, experimental studies have shown effects that are consistent with pathogenic factors in acute coronary events. Although the committee has confidence in the evidence of an association between chronic secondhand-smoke exposure and acute coronary events, the evidence on the magnitude of the association is less convincing, so the committee did not estimate that magnitude (that is, the effect size).

3. *Is it biologically plausible that a relatively brief (e.g., under 1 hour) secondhand smoke exposure incident could precipitate an acute coronary event? If yes, what is known or suspected about how this risk may vary based upon absence or presence (and extent) of preexisting coronary artery disease?*

There is no direct evidence that a relatively brief exposure to secondhand smoke can precipitate an acute coronary event; few published studies have addressed that question. The circumstantial evidence of such a relationship, however, is compelling. The strongest evidence comes from air-pollution research, especially research on PM. Although the source of the PM can affect its toxicity, particle size in secondhand smoke is comparable with that in air pollution, and research has demonstrated a similarity between cardiovascular effects of PM and of secondhand smoke. Some studies have demonstrated rapid effects of brief secondhand-smoke exposure (for example, on platelet aggregation and endothelial function), but more research is necessary to delineate how secondhand smoke produces cardiovascular effects and the role of underlying preexisting coronary arterial disease in determining susceptibility to the effects. Given the data on PM, especially those from time-series studies, which indicate that a relatively brief exposure can precipitate an acute coronary event, and the fact that PM is a major component of secondhand smoke, the committee concludes that it is biologically plausible for a relatively brief exposure to secondhand smoke to precipitate an acute coronary event.

With respect to how the risk might vary in the presence or absence of preexisting coronary arterial disease, it is generally assumed that acute coronary events are more likely to occur in people who have some level of preexisting disease, although that underlying disease is often subclinical. There are not enough data on the presence of pre-existing coronary arterial disease in the populations studied to assess the extent to which the absence or presence of such preexisting disease affects the cardiovascular risk posed by secondhand-smoke exposure.

4. *What is the strength of the evidence for a causal relationship between indoor smoking bans and decreased risk of acute myocardial infarction?*

The key intervention studies that have evaluated the effects of indoor smoking bans consistently have shown a decreased risk of heart attack. Research has also indicated that secondhand-smoke exposure is causally related to heart attacks, that smoking bans decrease secondhand-smoke exposure, and that a relationship between secondhand-smoke exposure and acute coronary events is biologically plausible. All the relevant studies have shown an association in a direction consistent with a causal relationship (although the committee was unable to estimate the magnitude of the association), and the committee therefore concludes that the evidence is sufficient to infer a causal relationship.

5. *What is a reasonable latency period between a decrease in secondhand smoke exposure and a decrease in risk of an acute myocardial infarction for an individual? What is a reasonable latency period between a decrease in population secondhand smoke exposure and a measurable decrease in acute myocardial infarction rates for a population?*

No direct information is available on the time between a decrease in secondhand-smoke exposure and a decrease in the risk of a heart attack in an individual. Data on PM, however, have shown effects on the heart within 24 hours, and this supports a period of less than 24 hours. At the population level, results of the key intervention studies reviewed by the committee are for the most part consistent with a decrease in risk as early as a month following reductions in secondhand-smoke exposure; however, given the variability in the studies and the lack of data on the precise timing of interventions, the smoking-ban studies do not provide adequate information on the time it takes to see decreases in heart attacks.

6. *What are the strengths and weaknesses of published population-based studies on the risk of acute myocardial infarction following the institution of comprehensive indoor smoking bans? In light of published studies' strengths and weaknesses, how much confidence is warranted in reported effect size estimates?*

Some of the weaknesses of the published population-based studies of the risk of MI after implementation of smoking bans are

- Limitations associated with an open study population and, in some cases, with the use of a small sample.
- Concurrent interventions that reduce the observed effect of a smoking ban.
- Lack of exposure-assessment criteria and measurements.
- Lack of information collected on the time between the cessation of exposure to secondhand smoke and changes in disease rates.
- Differences between control and intervention groups.
- Nonexperimental design of studies (by necessity).
- Lack of assessment of the sensitivity of results to the assumptions made in the statistical analysis.

The different studies had different strengths and weaknesses in relation to the assessment of the effects of smoking bans. For example, the Scottish study had such strengths as prospective design and serum cotinine measurements. The Saskatoon study had the advantage of comprehensive hospital records, and the Monroe County study excluded smokers. The population-based studies of the risk of heart attack after the institution of comprehensive smoking bans were consistent in showing an association between the smoking bans and a decrease in the risk of acute coronary events, and this strengthened the committee's confidence in the existence of the association. However, because of the weaknesses discussed above and the variability among the studies, the committee has little confidence in the magnitude of the effects and, therefore, thought it inappropriate to attempt to estimate an effect size from such disparate designs and measures.

7. *What factors would be expected to influence the effect size? For example, population age distribution, baseline level of secondhand smoke protection among nonsmokers, and level of secondhand smoke protection provided by the smoke-free law.*

A number of factors that vary among the key studies can influence effect size. Although some of the studies found different effects in different age groups, these were not consistently identified. One major factor is the size of the difference in secondhand-smoke exposure before and after implementation of a ban, which would vary and depends on: the magnitude of exposure before the ban, which is influenced by the baseline level of smoking and preexisting smoking bans or restrictions; and the magnitude of exposure after implementation of the ban, which is influenced by the extent of the ban, enforcement of and compliance with the ban, changes in social norms of smoking behaviors, and remaining exposure in areas not covered by the ban (for example, in private vehicles and homes). The baseline rate of acute coronary events or cardiovascular disease could influence the effect size, as would the prevalence of other risk factors for acute coronary events, such as obesity, diabetes, and age.

8. *What are the most critical research gaps that should be addressed to improve our understanding of the impact of indoor air policies on acute coronary events? What studies should be performed to address these gaps?*

The committee identified the following gaps and research needs as those most critical for improving understanding of the effect of indoor-air policies on acute coronary events:

- The committee found a relative paucity of data on environmental cardiotoxicity of secondhand smoke compared with other disease end points related to secondhand smoke, such as carcinogenicity and reproductive toxicity. Research should develop standard definitions of cardiotoxic end points in pathophysiologic studies (for example, specific results on standard assays) and a classification system for cardiotoxic agents (similar to the International Agency for Research on Cancer classification of carcinogens). Established cardiotoxicity assays for environmental exposures and consistent definitions of adverse outcomes of such tests would improve investigations of the cardiotoxicity of secondhand smoke and its components and identify potential end points for the investigation of the effects of indoor-air policies on acute coronary events.
- The committee found a lack of a system for surveillance of the prevalence of cardiovascular disease and of the incidence of acute coronary events in the United States. Surveillance of incidence and prevalence trends would allow secular trends to be taken into account better and to be compared among different populations to establish the effects of indoor-air policies. Although some national databases and surveys include cardiovascular end points, a national database that tracks hospital admission rates and deaths from acute coronary events, similar to the SEER database for cancer, would improve epidemiologic studies.
- The committee found a lack of understanding of a mechanism that leads to plaque rupture and from that to an acute coronary event and of how secondhand smoke affects that process. Additional research is necessary to develop reliable biomarkers of early effects on plaque vulnerability to rupture and to improve the design of pathophysiologic studies of secondhand smoke that examine effects of exposure on plaque stability.

- All 11 key studies reviewed by the committee have strengths and limitations due to their study design, and none was designed to test the hypothesis that secondhand-smoke exposure causes cardiovascular disease or acute coronary events. Because of those limitations and the consequent variability in results, the committee did not have enough information to estimate the magnitude of the decrease in cardiovascular risk due to smoking bans or to a decrease in secondhand-smoke exposure. A large, well-designed study could permit estimation of the magnitude of the effect. An ideal study would be prospective; would have individual-level data on smoking status; would account for potential confounders, including other risk factors for cardiovascular events (such as obesity and age), would have biomarkers of mainstream and secondhand-smoke exposures (such as blood cotinine concentrations); and would have enough cases to allow separate analyses of smokers and nonsmokers or, ideally, stratification of cases by cotinine concentrations to examine the dose–response relationship. Such a study could be specifically designed for secondhand smoke or potentially could take advantage of existing cohort studies that might have data available or attainable for investigating secondhand-smoke exposure and its cardiovascular effects, such as was done with the INTERHEART study. Existing studies that could be explored to determine their utility and applicability to questions related to secondhand smoke include the Multi-Ethnic Study of Atherosclerosis (MESA) study, the American Cancer Society's CPS-3, the European Prospective Investigation of Cancer (EPIC), the Framingham Heart Study, and the Jackson Heart Study. Researchers should clearly articulate the assumptions used in their statistical models and include analysis of the sensitivity of results to model choice and assumptions.

REFERENCES

Barone-Adesi, F., L. Vizzini, F. Merletti, and L. Richiardi. 2006. Short-term effects of Italian smoking regulation on rates of hospital admission for acute myocardial infarction. *European Heart Journal* 27(20):2468-2472.

Bartecchi, C., R. N. Alsever, C. Nevin-Woods, W. M. Thomas, R. O. Estacio, B. B. Bartelson, and M. J. Krantz. 2006. Reduction in the incidence of acute myocardial infarction associated with a citywide smoking ordinance. *Circulation* 114(14):1490-1496.

Bhatnagar, A. 2006. Environmental cardiology: Studying mechanistic links between pollution and heart disease. *Circulation Research* 99(7):692-705.

CDC (Centers for Disease Control and Prevention). 2009. Reduced hospitalizations for acute myocardial infarction after implementation of a smoke-free ordinance—city of Pueblo, Colorado, 2002–2006. *MMWR—Morbidity & Mortality Weekly Report* 57(51):1373-1377.

Cesaroni, G., F. Forastiere, N. Agabiti, P. Valente, P. Zuccaro, and C. A. Perucci. 2008. Effect of the Italian smoking ban on population rates of acute coronary events. *Circulation* 117(9):1183-1188.

Ellerbeck, E. F., S. F. Jencks, M. J. Radford, T. F. Kresowik, A. S. Craig, J. A. Gold, H. M. Krumholz, and R. A. Vogel. 1995. Quality of care for Medicare patients with acute myocardial infarction. A four-state pilot study from the cooperative cardiovascular project. *JAMA* 273(19):1509-1514.

Hamill, P. V. 1997. Re: "Invited commentary: Response to Science article, 'Epidemiology faces its limits.'" *American Journal of Epidemiology* 146(6):527-528.

He, J., S. Vupputuri, K. Allen, M. R. Prerost, J. Hughes, and P. K. Whelton. 1999. Passive smoking and the risk of coronary heart disease--a meta-analysis of epidemiologic studies. *New England Journal of Medicine* 340(12):920-926.

HEI (Health Effects Institute) Accountability Working Group. 2003. *Assessing the health impact of air quality regulations: Concepts and methods for accountability research. Communication 11.* Boston, MA: Health Effects Institute.

HHS (U.S. Department of Health and Human Services). 2006. *The health consequences of involuntary exposure to tobacco smoke: A report of the surgeon general.* Atlanta, GA: U.S. Department of Health and Human Services, Centers for Disease Control and Prevention, Coordinating Center for Health Promotion, National Center for Chronic Disease Prevention and Health Promotion, Office on Smoking and Health.

Hill, A. B. 1965. The environment and disease: Association or causation? *Proceedings of the Royal Society of Medicine* 58:295-300.

Juster, H. R., B. R. Loomis, T. M. Hinman, M. C. Farrelly, A. Hyland, U. E. Bauer, and G. S. Birkhead. 2007. Declines in hospital admissions for acute myocardial infarction in New York state after implementation of a comprehensive smoking ban. *American Journal of Public Health* 97(11):2035-2039.

Khuder, S. A., S. Milz, T. Jordan, J. Price, K. Silvestri, and P. Butler. 2007. The impact of a smoking ban on hospital admissions for coronary heart disease. *Preventive Medicine* 45(1):3-8.

Lemstra, M., C. Neudorf, and J. Opondo. 2008. Implications of a public smoking ban. *Canadian Journal of Public Health* 99(1):62-65.

Mills, N. L., H. Tornqvist, M. C. Gonzalez, E. Vink, S. D. Robinson, S. Soderberg, N. A. Boon, K. Donaldson, T. Sandstrom, A. Blomberg, and D. E. Newby. 2007. Ischemic and thrombotic effects of dilute diesel-exhaust inhalation in men with coronary heart disease. *New England Journal of Medicine* 357(11):1075-1082.

Morrow, D. A., E. M. Antman, L. Parsons, J. A. de Lemos, C. P. Cannon, R. P. Giugliano, C. H. McCabe, H. V. Barron, and E. Braunwald. 2001. Application of the TIMI risk score for ST-elevation MI in the National Registry of Myocardial Infarction 3. *JAMA* 286(11):1356-1359.

Pell, J. P., S. Haw, S. Cobbe, D. E. Newby, A. C. H. Pell, C. Fischbacher, A. McConnachie, S. Pringle, D. Murdoch, F. Dunn, K. Oldroyd, P. Macintyre, B. O'Rourke, and W. Borland. 2008. Smoke-free legislation and hospitalizations for acute coronary syndrome. *New England Journal of Medicine* 359(5):482-491.

Rogers, W. J., L. J. Bowlby, N. C. Chandra, W. J. French, J. M. Gore, C. T. Lambrew, R. M. Rubison, A. J. Tiefenbrunn, and W. D. Weaver. 1994. Treatment of myocardial infarction in the United States (1990 to 1993). Observations from the National Registry of Myocardial Infarction. *Circulation* 90(4):2103-2114.

Sargent, R. P., R. M. Shepard, and S. A. Glantz. 2004. Reduced incidence of admissions for myocardial infarction associated with public smoking ban: Before and after study. *BMJ* 328(7446):977-980.

Seo, D.-C., and M. R. Torabi. 2007. Reduced admissions for acute myocardial infarction associated with a public smoking ban: Matched controlled study. *Journal of Drug Education* 37(3):217-226.

Stranges, S., M. Cummings, F. P. Cappuccio, and M. Travisan. 2007. Secondhand smoke exposure and cardiovascular disease. *Current Cardiovascular Risk Reports* 1(5):373-378.

Teo, K. K., S. Ounpuu, S. Hawken, M. R. Pandey, V. Valentin, D. Hunt, R. Diaz, W. Rashed, R. Freeman, L. Jiang, X. Zhang, S. Yusuf, and I. S. Investigators. 2006. Tobacco use and risk of myocardial infarction in 52 countries in the INTERHEART study: A case-control study. *Lancet* 368(9536):647-658.

U.S. Public Health Service. 1964. *Smoking and health: Report of the Advisory Committee of the Surgeon General of the Public Health Service*. PHS Publication No. 1103. Washington, DC.

Vasselli, S., P. Papini, D. Gaelone, L. Spizzichino, E. De Campora, R. Gnavi, C. Saitto, N. Binkin, and G. Laurendi. 2008. Reduction incidence of myocardial infarction associated with a national legislative ban on smoking. *Minerva Cardioangiologica* 56(2):197-203.

Whincup, P. H., J. A. Gilg, J. R. Emberson, M. J. Jarvis, C. Feyerabend, A. Bryant, M. Walker, and D. G. Cook. 2004. Passive smoking and risk of coronary heart disease and stroke: Prospective study with cotinine measurement. *BMJ* 329(7459):200-205.

Appendix

Agendas of Public Meetings

FIRST PUBLIC MEETING
TUESDAY, DECEMBER 2, 2008
ROOM 202, KECK BUILDING
WASHINGTON, DC

- Welcome, Opening Remarks, and Introductions
  Lynn Goldman, M.D., M.P.H., Committee Chair
- Charge to the Committee
  Captain Matthew McKenna, M.D., M.P.H., Director, Office of
  Smoking and Health
  Dr. Darwin Labarthe, M.D., M.P.H., Ph.D., F.A.H.A., Director,
  Division for Heart Disease and Stroke Prevention
  Centers for Disease Control and Prevention
  Atlanta, Georgia
- Open Microphone and General Discussion
- Closing Remarks
  Lynn Goldman, M.D., M.P.H., Committee Chair

SECOND PUBLIC MEETING
FRIDAY, JANUARY 30, 2009
HUNTINGTON ROOM,
ARNOLD AND MABEL BECKMAN CENTER
100 ACADEMY DRIVE
IRVINE, CA

- Welcome, Opening Remarks, and Introductions
  Lynn Goldman, M.D., M.P.H., Committee Chair
- Smoking Ban Studies
  Stanton Glantz, Ph.D., University of California, San Francisco
- Overview of Surveillance Studies—Strengths, Weaknesses, and Capabilities
  Joel Kaufman, M.D., M.P.H., University of Washington, Seattle
- Open Microphone and General Discussion
- Adjourn Open Session